REDISCOVERED

of related interest

Arriving Late
The lived experience of women receiving a late autism diagnosis
Jodi Lamanna
ISBN 978 1 83997 510 3
eISBN 978 1 83997 511 0

Women and Girls on the Autism Spectrum, Second Edition
Understanding Life Experiences from Early Childhood to Old Age
Sarah and Jess Hendrickx
Foreword by Dr Judith Gould
ISBN 978 180501 069 2
eISBN 978 1 80501 070 8

This is Who I Am
The Autistic Woman's Creative Guide to Belonging
Andrea Anderson
ISBN 978 1 80501 015 9
eISBN 978 1 80501 016 6

Thumbsucker
An illustrated journey through an undiagnosed autistic childhood
Eliza Fricker
ISBN 978 1 83997 854 8
eISBN 978 1 83997 855 5

REDISCOVERED

A Compassionate and
Courageous Guide
For Late Discovered
Autistic Women
(and Their Allies)

CATHERINE ASTA

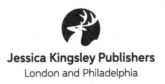

Jessica Kingsley Publishers
London and Philadelphia

First published in Great Britain in 2025 by Jessica Kingsley Publishers
An imprint of John Murray Press

2

Copyright © Catherine Asta 2025

The right of author name to be identified as the Author of the Work has been
asserted by her in accordance with the Copyright, Designs and Patents Act 1988.

Content warning: This book contains mention of
suicide, sexual abuse and victimization.

A CIP catalogue record for this title is available from the
British Library and the Library of Congress

ISBN 978 1 80501 150 7
eISBN 978 1 80501 151 4

Printed and bound in Great Britain by TJ Books Limited

Jessica Kingsley Publishers' policy is to use papers that are natural,
renewable and recyclable products and made from wood grown in
sustainable forests. The logging and manufacturing processes are expected
to conform to the environmental regulations of the country of origin.

Jessica Kingsley Publishers
Carmelite House
50 Victoria Embankment
London EC4Y 0DZ

www.jkp.com

John Murray Press
Part of Hodder & Stoughton Ltd
An Hachette Company

The authorised representative in the EEA is Hachette Ireland,
8 Castlecourt Centre, Dublin 15, D15 XTP3, Ireland (email: info@hbgi.ie)

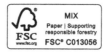

Contents

Acknowledgements 7

Introduction 10

1. Coming Home 12

2. Powering Progress 38

3. Our Sensory World 56

4. Our Emotional World 74

5. Our Cognitive World 86

6. The Places We Go to When the World Feels Too Much . . 105

7. When the Body Screams Enough 123

8. The Goldilocks Effect 139

9. Our Social and Relational World 155

10. Some of the Things We Don't Talk About Enough
    (But Need to Talk About More) 173

11. Workplaces We Thrive in 191

12. Your Rediscovered Tool Kit 209

Conclusion 230

References 232

Acknowledgements

This book is dedicated to all the people who have been my light in this journey into my new rediscovered world that I now know to be home.

My mum for being open to the many conversations I needed to have to understand myself more and for always advocating for me. For showing me what courage looks like and for accepting me for who I am.

To my eldest daughter who gave the 21-year-old me the gift of motherhood – and with it a purpose and focus in my life at a time when I needed it more than ever. She has been my driving force and, now an adult herself, is also my best friend. Thank you also for being my wing woman on the podcast and saying yes to my idea so we could bring The Late Discovered Club to life, and for taking care of me up this breast cancer mountain in all the ways you have. I'm thankful, feel privileged and so proud of the woman you have become and the life you are curating to continue your becoming.

My youngest daughter who is the gift that keeps on giving, helpfully uncovering a perspective and a viewpoint on myself I had never seen, nor considered before. Something I will be eternally grateful to her for facilitating in my own late discovery story. I have learnt so much from her and she inspires me to do this work, to help give the next generation the visibility I never had but needed and to keep deconstructing those stereotypes. I'm so proud of you for owning who you are and being courageously you, and reminding me to be courageously me. You radiate kindness and light and have such an infectious zest for life (and football).

I love you both so much and I have such a depth of gratitude that I was gifted the opportunity to be your mum and pour love and light into you both. And my stepchildren for the opportunity to share that love and light with you both too.

To my husband who despite the fact that we are separated, is co-parenting with me, and has been my sherpa up the breast cancer mountain – with me through the toughest parts. I hope this book gives you further insights and a greater understanding of why I needed to take and create that space and time for me, and that you continue the learning and the curiosity.

To my dad for the trip we went on together in 2023 to Copenhagen to reconnect and the stories we were able to share and the opportunity to understand each other on this rediscovered journey. For listening and being open and accepting of me, despite all the years we missed out on, and the emotional support and anchor you have been on my mountain climb.

To my editor Lynda Cooper for investing in my idea for this book and going at my pace.

To Melanie Kirkbride for giving me the gift of Vedic meditation. I will be forever grateful for the practice and for our connection. Even though you are now on the other side of the world I still feel our connection, and to Jillian Lavender for writing the book I needed, and at the time I needed to discover it.

Paris Ackrill for the lesson I needed in compassionate awareness and the discovery of somatic movement, the gift of profound rest, and the sanctuary and safe space you have held for me on my healing and rediscovered journey.

Jennifer Crichton for the inspiration and confidence you nurtured in me and my writing. Thank you for helping me step into my author era with self-belief. The column space opportunity you gave me was the reminder I needed.

My oncology team and the NHS for getting me up the breast cancer mountain so far so that this book could be written.

And all the guests who have allowed me the privilege to explore their late discovered stories on the podcast. Your courage and vulnerability in sharing your story has resonated with thousands of late discovered women across the world and has been the soothing balm I needed in my own rediscovered journey. Thank you for being the change.

To the people in The Late Discovered Club Community who shared their experiences in this book, I know the courage it takes to do this, and I am inspired by each and every one of you. Some of you wanted to remain anonymous in the contributions that you made, whilst others requested to be credited.

- Bex Dixon

- Lucy

- Sharon Martin

- Sophie Thomas

- Stephie

- Helen Hillman, 30 (late diagnosed autistic woman)

- Victoria Matthews Patel, coach and author

- M. She/her aged 53/diagnosed in 2022

- All the contributors who requested to remain anonymous

To Ed Jenneson and Kirsty Cullen-Campanelli for openly sharing your expertise. Your knowledge is received with the deepest gratitude.

To all the hundreds and hundreds of women I've worked with in therapy, in circles and those who have become part of The Late Discovered Club Community. Thank you for being brave and thank you for allowing me to be a small part of your stories.

And finally, all the autistic women who have paved the way before me, the trailblazers who have prepared the ground in this new world for me and others to follow. We see you and we give you our gratitude for opening the door to this brave new rediscovered world.

Introduction

From the point of autistic self-discovery there is a complete void of tailored post-discovery support that currently exists as the unravelling unfolds.

A lifetime of being misunderstood, the unseen struggles, the internalized shame and 'coming out' into a world where stigma and stereotypes exist, can make late discovery whilst life-affirming, also an incredibly discombobulating, lonely, imposter-inducing and equally painful place to find yourself in without the support or the community to guide you through it.

This is a book that will guide you from late discovered to rediscovered, to courageously seeking out and committing to a life that no longer under places your needs, but rather advocates those needs and champions you, and all from a strengths focused perspective, rooted in actually autistic experience, enveloped in compassion and understanding and layered through a therapeutic lens.

A book that every late discovered woman needs to read, and every ally and professional in your life needs to read too. I want this book to help you feel seen, heard, understood, empowered, with the self-permission and courage to take up your space and self-advocate for your needs, not as a different version of you, but as a *rediscovered* version of you, in the most self-compassionate, courageous and self-affirming way possible.

It's a book that I wish had existed when I needed that light and guided support, and I've written it in a way that feels intuitive and reflective of what I see, of the extensive work I've done in this area with hundreds and hundreds of late discovered women, and what I've experienced myself. And whilst it doesn't speak for all late discovered autistic women, it is rooted in autistic experience, including my own – experiences that until now, have never been given the airtime to be heard.

My hope is that this book empowers you on the journey to a rediscovered you, and that you too can find understanding, self-compassion and a sense of peace and acceptance for who you are – a coming home to yourself – recognizing the inner strengths that reside within you as well as the struggles you have and do experience, and are worthy and deserving of supporting.

Along with the self-permission and courage to start curating a life and an environment which enables you to show up and live your life going forwards aligned to your true authentic autistic self.

Because the story that you tell yourself about who you are matters.

You matter.

And this is your story – your **rediscovered story** to start writing.

It's time to come home to yourself.

Note: This book is written by an autistic woman and is rooted in over one hundred autistic experiences. It guides you from an autistic affirming perspective and uses identity-first language to help you understand you, advocate for you and to live a life aligned to your authentic autistic self. It does not use pathologizing language and aligns to the neurodiversity paradigm and utilizes a strengths- and compassion-based approach. It is not a diagnostic tool.

Content warning: Within the book references are made to suicide, sexual abuse and victimization.

CHAPTER 1

Coming Home

*Content warning: In this chapter I talk about suicide.

I wasn't actually diagnosed autistic until I was 44 years old. Like many in our late discovered community, it was motherhood that initiated the dawning discovery of my autistic self, and the unravelling of my undiscovered world as I knew it.

As I immersed myself into trying to make sense of this new world we found ourselves in, over a period of several years, I was, in parallel, attempting to make sense of my own world. Within the context of motherhood, there was a mirror that was being held up to me that I had never caught my reflection in until now. I consumed and absorbed everything I could find so that I could better support, accommodate and advocate, and create the environment our family needed, which in turn supported my own (unknown) needs.

I self-identified as autistic for many years, until I was eventually assessed by the NHS after several (unsupported) requests to my GP to be placed on the assessment pathway.

Autism wasn't a known or understood part of my world pre-discovery, yet here was the universe placing it right in front of me to not only make sense of it to help my family, but I now know to also help me rediscover myself, and to help others rediscover themselves too.

What I do know is that motherhood helpfully uncovered a perspective and a viewpoint on myself I had neither seen, nor considered before, and I am eternally grateful to my motherhood journey in facilitating this in my own late discovery story.

We all have a story

It's fair to say that I've experienced quite a lot in my 40+ years. I'm a late discovered multiply neurodivergent woman, who has experienced life, loss, trauma and adversity. I use the term 'multiply neurodivergent' because I also identify as being dyspraxic and ADHD.

I'm a breast cancer survivor too, diagnosed with an aggressive type of cancer just as I began writing this book. I've gone through months of chemotherapy (losing my hair in the process), surgery, radiotherapy and targeted treatment, and whilst I'm not quite at the top of the breast cancer mountain, it is very much in sight now and I hope that by the autumn/winter of 2024 that treatment will be complete and I'll be placing my colourful flag at the mountain summit, just as this book is published.

By means of a content warning, my writing is understandably influenced by this experience, as I wrote this book whilst climbing the breast cancer mountain, and I do draw on my cancer journey within the context of my autistic experience.

I've been a young single parent, and I've also been a parent navigating life in the blender that is blended family life. I embarked on motherhood all over again so have children across the age spectrum from seven to 23 years old, and I'm navigating new chapters relationally too and co-creating a different looking family construct in the process for me and my multiply neurodivergent children.

My work

Professionally, after graduating with a degree in psychology and sociology in the early 2000s, I then had a 12+-year career in Local Government Policy and Research, along with a good few years leading on National Strategy in the NHS and heading up Transformation for a large acute NHS Trust – all the while bringing up my daughter, who is now an adult herself.

In 2013, I made the decision to change career and studied alongside working full-time to qualify as a psychotherapist.

By late 2015 I had created my 'Bringing Sparkle Back Therapy' as a judgement-free space, full to the brim of compassion. It was my solution to something I had been looking for all my adult life but had yet to find. Since then, I've been a part of hundreds of women's stories and spent thousands of hours in the therapy room, and I embarked on further study with a master's in psychology, which I graduated from with Merit in 2022.

Pre-discovery, autism for me was something that was so far off my radar that I couldn't have even explained to you 'what' autism was. Autism wasn't something I studied in my undergraduate degree in psychology 25 years ago and it wasn't something that was on the curriculum when I trained to be a psychotherapist a decade ago.

The first time autism was really introduced to me in a professional context was back in 2020 when I embarked on my psychology masters, a conversion course so that I could springboard onto doctoral study, although, even then, it was in the context of a broad 'developmental psychology' module.

However, over the last few years my specialism has further focused into helping and supporting late discovered autistic women to rediscover themselves in a compassionate and courageous way through my 1:1 therapy, group circles, my podcast, community and hopefully through this book and the future books that I will write.

In 2022, I created 'The Late Discovered Club' Podcast with my eldest daughter Caty (as editor) to help give late discovered autistic women and marginalized groups a voice, deconstruct stereotypes and give the next generation visibility of autistic women and people. I wanted to create a space where our voices could be heard, and where our stories could become the lights of hope on someone else's dark runway.

The podcast has an ever-growing global community in over 120 countries and was ranked the number one podcast for 'Female Autism' in the world by FeedSpot in 2023.

As the podcast has grown, a community has organically developed around it. In addition to our Instagram community, we have a membership community with an online mighty community space where members can connect and we have a small, but growing number of community partners and champions supporting our work.

I lead and facilitate a six-week post discovery group circle online with people joining from across the world, as well as hosting events and conversations.

I'm also a consultant and speaker on all things women, autism and mental health, guest lecturing at UCL and co-authoring a chapter in a book published by Routledge in November 2024 on what neuro-inclusive therapy looks like in practice.

Since 2023 I've been co-training over 250 community and adult inpatient mental health professionals on what trauma informed and patient centered care looks like for autistic people as part of the NHS National Autism Trainer Programme.

I am listed in the Top 50 Influential Neurodivergent Women in the UK 2023, and was recognized as an Advocate For Change in Gender Equality 2023.

I can see clearly now the rain has gone

My late discovery felt like someone had wiped a circle on a steamed-up windscreen for me to see, a windscreen I didn't even know needed wiping. I thought everyone struggled to see, but once I saw this new landscape and new world through that small circle there was no going back – no 'unseeing' it or myself. It was this newfound perspective that ultimately directed me on a path to painfully confront and explore the Catherine I thought I was for the last four and a bit decades. I was catapulted into this new landscape, very much alone, and it became painfully obvious to me that I had crafted and built a very elaborate mask to enable me to live in a world that really wasn't built for my brain, and it had become too heavy a survival strategy to maintain.

I was beyond exhausted from wearing that mask. I have since learned that stress (particularly the post-traumatic type) intensifies how I experience the world as an autistic woman.

Through my work, I see an almost universally experienced

correlation of trauma in late discovered autistic women – our trauma is so often multilayered and multi-faceted. The most shocking discovery is that I have yet to meet an autistic woman who hasn't experienced repeated traumas throughout their life; and I am no exception.

My late discovery was, without a doubt, the most discombobulating chapter in my story so far, but equally the most affirming and profound because it explained so much of what I'd struggled with and why. Now it all seems so blatantly obvious, yet I also understand *why* it took me so long to rediscover myself in this way, and why I needed a mirror holding up to me so that I could see the parts of me I'd somehow disconnected from reflected right back at me.

But I was definitely in a state of shock. *How had I managed to keep this fundamental part of who I am behind a mask for so long, why had I done that* and *why didn't anyone else see the struggles behind the mask?*

Despite the revelation, I felt incredibly small and alone as I was existentially confronted with navigating this new landscape in this new world. Whilst it felt like I had 'come home' as I walked this new path, nothing looked familiar to me, yet I found myself deeply connected with everything and everyone that I discovered. I felt seen, heard and understood in this new world I was exploring, and I began to realize that this was the brave new world I would be calling home.

I was coming home and there was no going back to the world I had left.

Lightbulb moments

There were many lightbulb moments for me during that period of discovery. One of those moments was realizing that not everyone finds eye contact uncomfortable, intense and overwhelming, and that they don't avoid it wherever possible, yet this has been my internal experience for as long as I can remember. I've learned to do it, and I do it, but find it awkward and intense; it's something that feels forced and unnatural to me, especially in those unscripted social moments.

As part of my autism assessment, my eldest daughter was able to contribute (given she's lived with me for over two decades) and she picked up that eye contact is something I either do massively, with eye contact that doesn't break and is intense, or I avoid it altogether. It's in the water cooler conversations, the school playground small talk, the appointments with health professionals, the polite exchanges with the checkout assistant, the bumping into people unexpectedly, the interactions with the people in the cafe as I order my coffee, the group situations when more than one set of eyes are on you. When people expect you to show up in a certain way – their neuronormative way – I have had to find a work around, a survival technique to mask all that uncomfortableness, awkwardness and sensory trauma I'm feeling inside, and to deal with the consequences later. In fact any situation where people are looking at me I find excruciatingly uncomfortable.

I realize now that what I experience is visual overwhelm. They say that our eyes are the windows to our soul, and my windows are hypersensitive. My neurology takes everything in, and it overwhelms my sensory and nervous system. Looking away, closing my eyes, dim lights, filtering with sunglasses, and not maintaining eye contact are my ways of minimizing the visual overwhelm I feel.

And in so many group situations in my life in environments where it's not safe to unmask, I have adapted by staying quiet, a spoken word shutdown, being the intent listener and question asker, not taking up my space, or speaking up even though I have so much I want to say. I have stayed under the radar wherever possible – the super-compliant, introverted version of Catherine. By default this has meant that I have tended to surround myself throughout my life with people who are the life and soul, giving others the centre stage, a 'social aid' in many situations for me. I find myself being the space holder for others – the quiet, smiling, low needs/low maintenance, always-together version of Catherine.

The number of parties, dinners, weddings and social events I've been at and haven't fully contributed my experience or opinions to the conversation. It means you are there, but people never really know who you are. And in almost all of those situations I've experienced extreme, severe gastro flare ups. I remember attending weddings as a guest, as well as my own wedding, where I spent the vast majority of the time locked in the disabled toilet because my gastrointestinal system was in turmoil, and dinner parties where I've had to excuse myself partway through to escape to the safety of the bathroom. The anxiety I felt in social situations showed up so obviously, yet I never made the connection until my late discovery. I always blamed it on the food I ate; I believed that it was the food that triggered these responses, but what I'm learning is that it's actually a very physical reaction to a situation that is overwhelming me.

I've crafted a life where I'm always the 'behind the scenes'; I'm the make-sure-everyone-is-ok type in those scenarios, the facilitator, the enabler, the space holder, the adept listener and soaker-upper, existing under the radar and behind a smile. In social settings, I'm forever on a quest to find that one person I can connect with, who can accommodate the connection depth I need. And the problem with living your life for four decades like that is that nobody ever actually sees the struggles, and it makes navigating group social situations something I would much rather avoid, and have avoided – the result of that has been never really feeling like I belong.

It's much easier to show up as the community builder and the facilitator. The one leading, as opposed to 'doing'. Never the one asking for help, always the one giving it. Making plenty of space for others to be vulnerable, yet never feeling like I can show my vulnerabilities myself or express what I might need.

The sidecar

It has felt like for a lot of my life that I've placed myself as a passenger in a sidecar, switching to the driving seat only when the environment and conditions are right. It's not about a lack of confidence, because my life is made up of multiple bold moves and courageous choices – rather it's about environments that are disabling for me.

With the *right* environments I thrive, I know this because I've been unconsciously curating those environments throughout my life out of sheer necessity; however, now I know *why* I need my world to feel 'just right' for me to thrive, and how and why making those adjustments and accommodations for myself are no longer a 'nice to do', or a 'should do' but a 'must do' – my body has screamed 'enough' to me.

As I write this book I'm also climbing the breast cancer mountain, determined that I will get to the top. Once I've conquered this mountain and I've placed my colourful flag at the top and got safely back down the mountain I will continue, with a more appreciable determination and commitment to live this second chance at life that I've been gifted in a more gentle and nurturing way, with a greater compassionate awareness towards myself and my now known needs.

No more hiding my struggles; I'll be saying no in greater quantities, and curating the space to focus on the things that soothe me, bring me joy and play to my strengths.

I also recognize how being in the world as an undiscovered autistic woman has created power imbalances and an inherent vulnerability in many of the relational and social aspects throughout my life, and during my late discovered journey I couldn't help but question whether that knowledge about 'who' I am earlier *might* have safeguarded me from some of the harm I've been exposed to throughout my life.

Would I have been able to advocate for myself and protect myself more from the harm I've experienced?

Late discovery is jam-packed full of these 'what if?' questions, which is what makes it such an exhausting process. No stone goes untouched, everything has to be re-examined through this new lens, until it makes sense. It's like living in a sliding doors multiverse, but one that everybody on the outside is completely oblivious to.

Late discovery

During my own late discovery I was lucky and incredibly privileged both that my parents are still here for me to have the conversations I needed to have with them about how I was as a child, and that they were both open and engaged in the many conversations I've had with them to help me make sense of myself through this newfound autistic lens.

However, I recognize that many on their late discovery journey will not have this access because they have no contact with their parents, or their parents are not open to having this conversation, or because their parents are no longer here. There are also people who won't feel comfortable having the conversation with their parents, perhaps because they do not want to upset or 'burden' their elderly parents with their discovery – especially given the generational gaps in knowledge, awareness and acceptance, and the cultural challenges that exist in some communities.

There is also the very real and understandable fear of outright rejection and invalidation, all of which create even more barriers to accessing a diagnosis when your developmental history is a key and central part to that process.

A late 70s child, I originate from working class roots, and I'm one of seven girls in my family (the middle child of three from my parents' first marriage). My mum described me as a highly sensitive child – sensitive to my environment, sensitive to pain, sensitive to illness, sensitive to people, and sensitive to the world around me. A 'serious and deep' child who often misinterpreted things that were said, who had a need for order and structure, who rarely misbehaved and was hypersensitive to getting things wrong.

My speech was delayed and I would point rather than talk, making up words if I couldn't say them. I developed my own language and way of communicating which my mum understood but others struggled with. As a child I would get my words jumbled up, and spent my early years in speech therapy. I struggled with my pronunciation, which still happens now, although I try my hardest to overcome that as much as I can, and I struggle to recall words, or get them in the right order. I have to work really hard on my speech, and spoken word shutdown, scripting and solitude seeking I now recognize is often the outcome of my internalized overwhelm.

I spent a lot of time in my own world as a younger child, refusing at some points to go to school, preferring to play on my own. I was a child who was bullied – physically and verbally – throughout my childhood and as I moved into high school.

I was besieged by nightmares and night terrors throughout my childhood which have continued through into adulthood, and I have a brain that never stops and struggles to switch off for sleep – it is *always* firing, even whilst I'm asleep I dream so vividly, it feels like I have an overabundance of neurons that are constantly firing and connecting. That's how I imagine my brain – lit up and always on, always ready to go and hypersensitive to the world around me.

In fact, it was a dream about finding a lump in my breast that made me check my breasts one June morning in 2023. I had known that something wasn't right in the months prior to this dream, but my doctor, via a telephone consultation, put my symptoms down to perimenopause and sent me away with a few websites to explore around menopause. Two weeks after the dream, on 4th July 2023, I was diagnosed with a Grade 3 aggressive type of breast cancer that had already spread to my lymph nodes. Here was my own body alerting me to the fact something wasn't right. Yet so often we are not listened to and misbelieved when it comes to our health and our bodies.

I recognize that my brain works at 100 mph – it sees endless possibilities, solutions to problems, words as data, clarity in complexity, patterns in people's stories and is full to the brim of creativity and ideas. I now have an ideas journal, a place where I dump my gushing waterfall of next big ideas, and I have bought far too many domain names for businesses I'm never going to start but there's something about the dopamine high my brain gets from idea generation and creating something new.

I don't have an attention deficit, rather an abundance of attention I want to give to multiple things. It's an internal hyperactivity – my brain never stops. Finding an outlet in which to direct that energy and attention is an ever-present challenge – I wake up each day wanting to both savour the world and save it, which I attribute to being AuDHD (autistic with a generous helping of ADHD). Anecdotally what I have seen in my work, and in the stories we explore on the podcast, is that ADHD is a common co-occurrence for many in the late discovered autistic community. Whilst I've not been formally assessed for ADHD, during my autism assessment ADHD and dyspraxia were noted in my report as co-occurring conditions.

I also have a really big fear of the dark and I have an overactive imagination when it comes to the dark and watching scary movies, along with a petrifying fear of dogs, fish and pretty much most animals.

The stereotype that all autistic girls and women love animals is not my experience. For me, the unpredictability of not knowing how an animal might behave puts me in a heightened state of fear. People, on the other hand, I've been studying my whole life and they are much more predictable and human behaviour more understandable.

Growing up

As a child, I would seek the safety of retreating into my own world, not because of a 'deficit' in my ability to socialize, rather because the world can feel too much when your sensory system reacts in the way mine does to the world. Spending time in an environment that feels sensory-neutral equals safety, and I crave that solitude to recalibrate and decompress.

I had many conversations with my mum about growing up in the context of my late discovery, and one of those conversations helped us both to understand why I had big overspills at school. That conversation also helped me to understand why I would so often try to abscond and run away from situations at school and at home where there was too much sensory input (and find myself hiding under tables, beds and trees to block the external world out) or I thought that I'd done something wrong, not followed the rules correctly or made a mistake. It also helped me understand why navigating friendships was so very complex.

I was that child who would pack my belongings into a bin liner and run away from home when the world felt too much. I would always head for the woods in our local park and sit under the safety of the branches of the strong and sturdy trees, or lose myself in the oil seed rape fields that grew opposite our home. Looking back, I just needed a space where my highly sensitive nervous system could feel regulated, and I found that nature and solitude were instant sensory soothers for me.

As an adult, I found it was my running shoes and a bumbag. I'd take myself off in times of emotional distress and overwhelm and run for as long as I could, and as far as I could. That *flight* response has been my go-to for the last four decades and it has gotten me out of many situations in my life that have caused me distress, harm and overwhelm. It has, however, meant that I've found myself having to start again multiple times in my life; I can't tell you where 'home' is because I've lived in so many and that is an exhausting way to have to live your life.

My mum talked about the difficulties I experienced at school, which the school attributed to adverse events in my childhood but were actually due to the trauma of being in a school environment which was challenging because I was an (undiagnosed) autistic person. Without an understanding back then, I had no frame of reference as to why or what might help, so I tried my hardest to fit in, but I never really got it right.

I didn't fit and I didn't belong.

During my late discovery, I pondered what it was about me that my peers found so unpalatable and concluded that at some point in my childhood I began to avoid, or heavily mask in the situations that might trigger overspills or made my differences stand out – I internalized it all and sat firmly under the radar in the hope I might fit in.

I remember the crushing humiliation of being ghosted at high school by a group of friends, isolated and unsure as to why everyone had stopped talking to me. High school was a particular pain point for me, I was bullied physically by one particular group of older girls, never in school, always on my way to and from school when I was on my own, and despite my academic abilities, I began to disengage with school and bunk off whenever the opportunity arose.

Alcohol as social armour

As a young teen I discovered alcohol which became another fundamental part of my masking armour. This in turn created an added vulnerability, and got me into many situations that put me at risk and opened a door to harm as a young woman.

My teenage years were a lonely time; in addition to feeling like I didn't belong in the world, I had also been separated from my sisters after divorce hit our family hard when I was nine years old. Overnight, everything I had known changed – my home, my school, my community – and I no longer had the cushion of my older and younger sisters or my wider family network to help me navigate the world. I eventually lost contact with my dad for a significant period of time too.

I visualize this chapter in my life as a tremor line, the kind you see post-earthquake, where the landscape changes forever, yet at the time I didn't have the words or the ability to express any of the emotion or loss I was feeling in the way that was expected. Autism added another layer to that trauma and loss, and understanding that really helped me understand myself, and why I struggled so much at that point in my life. The lens of autism enabled me to show the younger version of me a level of compassion I've been unable to extend to myself until now. My mind creating the visual of an earthquake tremor line tells me now how significant and profound that period of my life was.

In early 2023, I took a trip to Copenhagen with my dad to reconnect with him and we talked of the many emotional overspills I had on holidays and days out, including the post-divorce Florida holiday my dad took my sisters and me on in 1989, when I got sunstroke because I couldn't bear the feel or the smell of the sun cream on my skin so washed it off, only for us all to be holed up in a hotel room for days because I was fainting and ill from sunstroke and with painfully blistered skin. I struggled whenever I was away from home, and seemed to be the only one struggling in these situations – the 'over-sensitive' 'drama queen' 'demanding' Catherine.

Our family moved to a different county just as I was beginning my GCSEs, which meant starting another new school and I remember the emotional outburst I had at the thought of moving schools and starting 'again' as a teenager. Being almost six foot tall, clearly autistic (but unaware), with a different accent and a distinctively different style to my peers, it's fair to say that the new girl fitted in even less. As soon as the bell rang for lunch I retreated to the safety of my home where I would have the same lunch of my beige, safe food on repeat.

I went to an average state secondary school. I was academically very bright, but their aspirations for me were low. The 15-year-old me wanted to be a journalist, I was fascinated by people and their stories – but my work experience was in a shop. Ultimately my response was that I disengaged with being excited about my life and could not see my future potential. Knowing how my mind works now, I can see why and how I disengaged – being under-stimulated with that abundance of neuronal energy and activity that resides in my head is as soul destroying as being over-stimulated.

I know that neither my parents nor my teachers knew what autism was, or how it presents in girls back in the 70s and 80s. I know they wouldn't have seen it, because our understanding of autism is largely based on the narrative we've been fed historically from autism research on mainly white (cisgender) males, which has categorically and systematically failed to explore the inner lived experience of autistic girls, women and marginalized groups, resulting in a gender-biased diagnostic criteria and a stereotype to match.

I also know that my parents did their best under their own set of (extremely) challenging circumstances. They had to parent in the dark, without any helpful neurodivergent framework, lens or support that I have access to as a parent. I have a much more compassionate and deeper understanding for my parents knowing what I know now, and a lot of love for them both.

Closing the book on my story

The blindfold coming off and back-cataloguing my life through a completely different lens has been challenging, as has the loss I experienced as I began to realize the extent of the missed knowledge and opportunities for adaptations, adjustments and nurturing of my strength that might have resulted in my life not feeling so difficult. Perhaps I would not have quit my A Levels, left home at 18, and attempted to take my own life by suicide in my late teens.

Thankfully I survived to write the next chapter of my story, the one where I became a mum at 21 to my daughter Caty, and channelled the drive and focus she gave me to get myself into university, so I could support the life I knew my daughter deserved, and live a life I knew I was capable and deserving of.

I'm pretty sure that I only survived university without dropping out because I had to combine study with looking after a small human. There was no time or opportunity to be sociable, make friends, or to be on campus longer than I needed to be, and the vast majority of my study was done at home, at night whilst Caty slept.

My suicide attempt at 19 years old was the ultimate flight response and self-harm. Despite a psychological assessment in the hospital nobody took the time to ask me 'why?'. Here was an opportunity to speak to a professional about my many struggles, but all they wanted to know was that I wouldn't attempt it again.

I wasn't given any preventative measures or a safety plan and was discharged home alone. That attempt became a shameful secret I kept hidden from everyone, including myself, until decades later when I was able to confront the painful truth I'd stashed away from even my own conscious view.

The emotional submarine

With all the newfound knowledge and insights, and now an autism lens to help frame four decades of experiences 'that label' helped me and gave me permission to be curious, enabling me access to a whole other level of self-understanding and uncover previously repressed experiences I had packed off on an emotional submarine full of pain points, deep into the darkest of oceanic depths.

The emotional submarine was an act of self-protection from the many painful experiences which had triggered so much internalized shame and humiliation, until I gave it permission to surface, saying 'Hey, I'm here and I'm now ready to be unpacked'.

It felt as though as soon as I opened the heavy, air-tight door to that submarine, the unpacking had to happen, and it did. Memories flowed and past painful experiences were given the airtime they so clearly needed, I had to confront them – I was ready to confront them through an autistic lens. But that unpacking brought a lot of sadness bubbling to the surface – I discovered that this was grief work.

I realized, as I navigated and guided my way through the contents on board this surfaced submarine, that my differences were never seen or understood in the era I grew up in – a time in the history of autism when we knew so little about autism and girls. I was born in 1979, and the concept of a 'spectrum' was only introduced a few years after that by Dr Lorna Wing. Just a decade before I was born, Dr Bruno Bettleheim, a psychoanalyst and a prominent figure in the field of autism research at the time, suggested that autism was a psychological 'disorder' caused by maternal coldness and a lack of maternal bonding. His 'refrigerator mother' theory positioned itself as a central theory to autism with his book, *The Empty Fortress*, published in 1967 further popularizing what we now know is a harmful and outdated theory. But his theory will have no doubt shaped a generation to believe that mothers were to blame, that autism was psychological rather than neurodevelopmental, echoes of which still reverberate in the 2020s in the pathological paradigm of disorder over the neurodiversity paradigm of difference. Is there any wonder then that there were no autistic women role models for me growing up?

The family trauma and adverse experiences I had lived through made the experience even more complex so I did for myself what I would do for anyone else – I allowed myself the space and the time to sit and acknowledge those newly-surfaced feelings, to mourn the loss of what I needed but couldn't ask for as a child and a young adult, and I gave myself the acceptance that I have spent my life searching for and the permission to embrace my authentic self.

During this process of late discovery, I recognized that, despite a toolbox full of therapeutic approaches and a 25-year deeply-focused interest on psychology and human behaviour, I needed support from others to help me explore myself, and I needed to find some new tools to help me connect with myself.

Like many women, I first reached out for help to my GP only to be told via text that I didn't meet the referral criteria for my local autism and ADHD pathway, which felt deeply invalidating. Having had the courage to say I needed some help, only to find myself locked out of a pathway that was supposed to help me, I felt very isolated. This is why self-identifying is absolutely valid, it's so often the *only* way. It's not about jumping on a bandwagon or watching a TikTok video and one day simply deciding that you are autistic. Rather, it's the result of being excluded because of your gender, from a government-funded system of support that doesn't see or understand autistic women and those from marginalized groups. The gender gap here, and the many many stories I hear about exclusion, is a shocking gender health inequality in our modern-day NHS. I wasn't sure what I needed or where I could access support as a self-identifying late discovered autistic woman, and in the absence of being seen, heard and understood with my new identity I felt I had no choice but to do the late discovery work myself.

I later went back to my GP and requested again to be referred for an assessment, only this time I was listened to, and eventually received an NHS autism diagnosis several years later. But throughout those years between being denied access to the assessment pathway and my eventual diagnosis I was still autistic. I was still struggling. I wasn't seen or believed and the heaviness of exploring my autistic self was exhausting. For several years I dived so deeply into trying to understand myself that it was all I thought about and all I wanted to talk about. It utterly consumed me. When my assessor asked me how I felt when she gave me my diagnosis I said I felt a sense of 'peace'. For this is no longer discovery work, it's now a rediscovered journey in courageously and compassionately coming home to myself and being at peace in this new world.

There was (and still is) very little therapy offered in the mainstream for this type of late discovery work. During my late discovery phase I personally wasn't looking for someone to validate what I knew about myself, or to help me make sense of my life through an allistic lens, or to give me coping mechanisms, or to help me reframe my thinking with a group course of CBT, or shift my behaviour. I definitely didn't need medicating because I wasn't depressed, yet a prescription of antidepressants was indeed the *only* help that I was actually offered.

Autistic enlightenment

What I needed was the space and time to explore myself and to be curious through this newfound autistic enlightenment. To offer myself the opportunity to be strengths- and compassion-focused, rather than deficit-led, and to understand my struggles and give them the acknowledgment and the acceptance they've always needed through a trauma-informed, experience-sensitive lens.

It felt like I'd already watched a film, and now I was going back to the beginning to rewatch it, to rediscover a different version, and this time I'd be noticing all the nuanced parts I never had the first time round. In the absence of a guide or someone to hold my hand through this, I took all my knowledge and insights and experience as a therapist, and what I already understood about myself, and guided myself through my own late discovery.

My beautiful autistic mind enabled me to imagine there was a rediscovered version of me, sitting with the late discovered me in the dark, guiding me and lighting up the way to 'coming home' unsure of what I would discover, but with a sense this was work I had to begin and that I was ready to start.

My trifecta of self-discovery tools

There was a powerful trifecta of tools that helped me rediscover myself, and the caveat here is that they were tools that I found worked *for me*. I was intuitively drawn to the power of these tools that, when combined, helped me to understand my autistic self.

Journaling

I found the process of writing things down, drawing pictures and connecting things – memories, thoughts, reflections, past experiences – so powerful. Through writing, narrating and reflecting on my own story, I had real moments of complete and utter clarity and self-knowing.

My journal bore the brunt of this unravelling and unpacking. I found journaling such a therapeutic process; there were plenty of 'aha' moments, but also a lot of sadness for having to navigate life for over four decades without the knowledge I now have and with the constant questions of 'what did I do wrong?', 'why don't I fit?' or 'why does my brain never stop?'.

It's a journal I regularly go back to because as I wrote those words, asked the questions, and drew the mind maps and pictures to connect the dots, I was rediscovering myself in real time, and there is something so potent and significant about what I discovered when I allowed myself the time and space to unpack my mind and to ask the questions.

Vedic meditation

Second, I discovered Vedic meditation. I was clearly seeking something out that could access a deeper, unconscious level and was craving peace and calm, because my mind works at lightning speed and never stops.

I read the book *Why Meditate, Because it Works* (Lavender, 2021) which introduced me to the concept of Vedic sound meditation. This led me to discover a wonderful Australian woman, Melanie, co-founder of 'The Soft Road' in my hometown, we connected and she taught me how to meditate the Vedic way.

Vedic meditation comes from 'the Veda, the ancient body of knowledge from India. The Veda is the source of yoga, meditation, and Ayurvedic medicine and is the basis of all Eastern philosophy' (The London Meditation Centre, 2024).

I was a little apprehensive about starting, having convinced myself that there would be absolutely no way my mind would quieten itself to meditate for 20 minutes, twice a day, every day. But the benefit of Vedic meditation (and I'm sure why it works so well for my 'always on' mind) is that you are given a mantra, a sound that you repeat in your head, and it's this mantra that quiets the mind.

And as my mind settled it began to create movement to the sound in my mind – from observing waves on a beach, to being sat on a swing. I noticed that my mind was creating movement that I found deeply meditative, movement that enabled me to access a part of myself I've never visited before. In my first session Melanie guided me, and I meditated for 20 minutes to my sound mantra. In that time I felt such a profound connection to myself, my mind took me to a place of complete peace and happiness, and I had an intense wave of emotion.

My mind was taking me to such descriptive, visual places, places I've never visited before, but that I could see myself in, and water was always present. After that first session I felt peaceful and content, and with a newfound connection to myself and my inner world I can honestly say I've never felt before. When we talk about dialling down our nervous system, and dialling up our relaxation response, this was it in practice for me.

Vedic meditation is known as the 'bliss technique' and after my very first session I described it as though I'd just had a 20-minute blissful endorphin bath full to the brim of serotonin, dopamine and oxytocin – it really was that good! For me, the combination of a sound for my mind to focus on, my need for calm and my visual-picture-thinking mind is a powerful outlet for me to access and process my emotions, something I realize I struggle to do. Through my meditation I unlocked and was able to process a lifetime of unresolved loss, and found it was a powerful tool in which to help me make sense of how I feel and also to find clarity in struggles I was facing. I re-emerged from my sessions with a newfound insight and perspective I'd previously not had access to.

And I think that must be the secret to how this becomes such an effortless daily practice. Think about it, we search for those endorphins in so many external things and pleasure-seek beyond ourselves, yet they exist within us, and meditation for me is a way to tap into those blissful endorphins. It's something I now can't imagine not being a part of life.

There is little research out there around the benefits of Vedic meditation for the autistic mind, however, research by (Sequeria & Ahmed, 2012) suggested that it may be 'an effective intervention for autism due to its documented capacity to reduce anxiety and may be a relatively simple practice to teach autistic individuals'. It is clear, however, that more research is needed to determine whether it is both feasible and beneficial for autistic individuals.

Community

Third: community. Finding other people like me, discovering shared experiences, and applying autistic frames around those experiences mattered. Community provided me with information and insights I'd never been privy to before. It made me feel seen and understood.

I found a sense of community and belonging through the many books, blogs, stories, media and social posts I consumed and saw myself reflected in – all authored by actually autistic people. And I've seen first-hand how bringing together small groups of late discovered women and people in our circle peer support group programmes and using our stories as a way of connecting has such a powerful effect on their late discovery journey too. Seeing ourselves in others, relating to experiences, hearing someone articulate something you have also felt, there is so much power in our stories.

Narrative psychology and peer support are powerful therapeutic tools that we need to embed more into post discovery/post-diagnostic support services.

In parallel to my late discovery process my tolerance and masking ability became harder and harder to maintain and enforce, and I had a sense that I was becoming more autistic, when in fact it was there all along. I had this vivid awareness that I had been masking my way through life and situations, and began to question my why and for whom – it was an unravelling like no other.

I found that there was a distinct lack of community and lens for late discovered women – our voices were not being heard, and our experiences not on anyone's radar, and so I began to build the community, and the autistic inclusive support and frameworks I could see were so obviously needed, but so evidently lacking.

The Late Discovered Club was my solution to this.

Rediscovered

And as I walked on this path of my own late discovery, I began to rediscover myself, accepting myself for who I am, self-identifying as an openly autistic woman and tentatively and gently disclosing the new 'rediscovered' version of myself. It felt like taking a pumice stone to a lifetime of shame, but the fear of not belonging and rejection in 'coming out' was also ever present – not knowing how people would respond to this life changing discovery, or indeed how applying such a pre-loaded stigmatized label to myself would affect me and my business, a business I've worked really hard to build.

- Would people's biases and judgements cancel me?

- Would people look at me and treat me differently?

- Would people question my ability to be a good therapist, given the myth that if you are autistic you can't possibly have empathy (along with all the other deficit-based myths people have been fed)?

- Would people distance themselves from me?

- Would people encourage me to keep this newfound knowledge about myself hidden?

- Would people be accepting of me?

Some of the responses were 'but you don't look autistic' or 'but you're too successful to be autistic'; others questioned 'why I'd want to give myself that label', or suggested I must have 'the high-functioning type'.

For some it confirmed what they knew, but the vast majority didn't really say anything, good or bad, and they didn't really want to know, understand or acknowledge, perhaps from a place of not really understanding what autism is, or even knowing the 'right' thing to say.

Autism doesn't have a 'look'.

I am an autistic woman who experiences and feels the world deeply, in every sense. My sensitivity, empathy, sensual and emotional thermostat is dialled up high, and that means that the world can feel too much, and I have big emotions that often become overwhelming, but others don't see that because it happens internally and the overspill and shutdown happens out of sight.

I have a highly sensitive sensory, immune, digestive, tissue and nervous system and the ability to deep dive for days, months, years and decades into things I have a passion for. I have a persistent drive for autonomy and a powerful and visual creative mind that is always existentially searching for depth and meaning.

I find comfort and safety in order, predictability and structure and have a pervasive need for space and solitude. I'm profoundly connected to nature, highly attuned somatically to my body, find joy in people's stories and building communities, need time to process and sense make, and find scripting a safety net to communicating verbally.

I've had to find elaborate and exhausting inner work-arounds and mask my way through life, and I categorically cannot, and will not, ever go back to living my life with only *that* view out of the windscreen. I am unable to go back to living my life that way. As I stepped into this new brave rediscovered world I knew that there was no going back. My newfound knowledge I now had about myself changed everything. There is a clear distinction between undiscovered autistic me and rediscovered me.

Understanding my struggles, and giving them the airtime and acceptance they've always needed (and deserved), has meant I can make empowering choices and adapt my life around my needs (something I realized I've been subconsciously doing throughout my life). It means I can seek out adjustments where I need them, and that I can focus on nurturing my strengths, rather than constantly pressing the override button on my nervous system to fit in.

As I have begun to delicately peel back the layers of the mask I've had to wear, I'm definitely living and experiencing my life in a more sensory friendly way: lowering the demands I place on myself, working with what's in the tank, dialling up the parts of me I've spent a lifetime dialling down, embracing my existential pull for depth, curiosity and creation, re-evaluating, simplifying, space making, self-advocating without any apologies, really leaning into what brings me joy and curating the environment I know I need to enable me to thrive.

It has also meant huge dollops of self-compassion, of being able to relate to myself in way that is forgiving, accepting and loving, and a lot of painful, but necessary change and difficult decisions to begin seeking out and committing to a life that no longer underplaces my needs, but rather advocates and champions those needs.

Coming home to myself

My late discovery signalled a new beginning for me as a 40-something woman. Coming home to myself meant showing up for myself in a way I've never been able to, or known how to before.

It meant a lot of self-forgiveness and finding an acceptance that others won't find this 'rediscovered' unmasked version of Catherine more/less palatable than the masked version of me. I've concluded that actually that's ok, because this next chapter in my life whilst I've been simultaneously climbing this breast cancer mountain is about embracing the rediscovered me, and allowing myself to design a life that allows me to be seen, heard and understood, with me and my needs as the headline, not as a tiny footnote.

And whilst there's a story of loss that comes with all of this, there is also the duality of new beginnings, and an excitement for what my life with this new perspective now guiding me is going to look and feel like. I'm a firm believer and an advocate of the dual process model of grief, of how the circle of grief and loss can sit alongside the circle of being action focused and forward-looking, and that somewhere in between those two circles lies the everyday living that we do.

And I realized in my own coming out that some people were, or are, in your life with a version of you that no longer exists. Others are here for the version of you that exists now; some will grow with you, and others won't.

And there are people who you have yet to meet. People who will get a version of you nobody else ever has – the version of you that is forever growing and learning and experiencing.

The rediscovered version.

And once I'd made that discovery, rather than continuing to swim against the tide, constantly feeling adrift at sea without an anchor point or dry land in the distance, I instead made the decision to immerse myself, my whole self into no longer trying to 'fit' into a world that wasn't built for the way I experience it, and giving myself the self-permission to be me.

- Understanding my struggles and strengths.

- Accommodating my differences.

- Advocating for my needs.

- Nurturing my strengths.

- Adapting in light of my struggles.

- Seeking out the environments I can thrive in.

- Placing myself in the centre of my own frequency circle when it comes to self-regulation and self-attunement.

- I am still me, but I'm not 'that' me anymore.

- I am rediscovered.

As a friend said to me, your autistic discovery is the Japanese 'Kintsugi' gold in the bowl. A discovery that isn't something to be ashamed of, despite the societal stigma that exists, but something rather that is illuminating, and shines a light on the beautiful way that your mind sees and experiences the world.

And this book is going to help you navigate that path of late discovery too, because...

- It's not just the late discovery that you are autistic.

- It's how late discovery validates decades of both felt and known difference, yet momentarily eclipses our sense of self and the darkness that ensues as you begin this rediscovery journey into self.

- It's the inability to continue living life the way you were pre-discovery.

- It's the 'how to' shed the layers upon layers of the mask you've had to wear and the fear of what lies beneath.

- It's all the parts of you that you've had to dial down.

- It's the lifetime of shame that you've carried.

- It's figuring out who you are, what you need, what you struggle with, how you strength nurture and how to stop pressing override on your nervous system. (It might be the first time that you've heard the phrase 'strength nurture' in this book, and it's a phrase I will refer to throughout. Strength nurturing essentially means getting to know what your strengths are, and then finding a way of integrating them into your daily life. Learning how to express them, and how you can make them a central part of your world.)

- It's the people who won't (and don't) want to understand this rediscovered version of you.

- It's the people who you thought might be allies who ghost and disappear.

- It's the relationships that change and can't or (won't) evolve or accommodate your needs.

- It's the boundaries you have to create and the apologies you stop giving for being you.

- It's the responses you get to the unmasked version of you.

- It's the need to find a place of belonging, a community of acceptance, a collective who get it, and who get you.

- It's all the ends it signals, and the new beginnings your late discovery creates to living your life authentically and aligned to your needs, with the acceptance and realization of who you are.

Because the story that you tell yourself about who you are matters. You matter.

And this is your story – your **rediscovered story** to start writing. It's time to come home to yourself.

CHAPTER 2

Powering Progress

Before I take you on the journey of rediscovery, I couldn't write this book without including a chapter which sets out the context and lays bare the shocking gender gap when it comes to late discovered autism and women's health, and the progress that we need to collectively power with our collective voices to narrow that inequality gap.

Allyship

My hope is that this book not only helps present and future late discovered autistic women to rediscover themselves in a self-compassionate and courageous way, but that this is a book you can gift to your friends and loved ones, to your boss and your colleagues, to your GP and health professionals, to the SENCOs in your children's schools, to your therapist – to anyone in your life who needs to understand the inside stories of an invisible neuro minority of women and who wants to become an ally.

And it's a book that parents and family members of autistic girls need in their lives too.

This book couldn't have been written without the valued contributions from the many women who came forward from our Late Discovered Club Community who wanted to share their rich inner world with you the reader.

These are stories and experiences that have never been heard or shared before from autistic women spanning seven decades and over 100 of these experiences are weaved into each chapter of this book, credited how they expressed they wanted to be credited.

Their experiences bring this book to life, and I will be forever grateful to those women who consented to being interviewed by me during the spring/summer of 2023.

Why this book and why now?

Late discovery at the point of motherhood was my anchor point, and it's a recurrent feature in the autistic women's stories that I've heard. Many people realize they are autistic later in life when their children or their grandchildren, nieces, nephews or wider family members go through the diagnostic process.

There's something about seeing yourself in the house of mirrors that your child or family member holds up to you which enables you to see yourself in a way and from a perspective you never have before. As you learn more about your child or family member, you begin to understand more about yourself in the process. There's nothing like going through the process of an autism assessment with your child or grandchild for the penny to drop that their challenges and struggles are the same challenges and struggles that you experienced, except now you have a narrative and frame of reference to put to that experience.

And then there are the women in our community who describe menopause and perimenopause as the point when 'the wheels start to fall off'; for many women, menopause is the point of their autistic discovery.

There are also late discovered women in our community who struggle at those transition points of university, work and motherhood, many of whom have collected several (mis) diagnoses of mental health conditions along the way, or have experienced a mental health crisis, suffered breakdowns, or have crashed out of jobs, education and work due to burnout before stumbling across their autism discovery.

We hear so much from health professionals, within our communities, in the media and amongst our families and friends about how late discovery can't be a thing, that if we've got this far then we really can't have struggled that much, or that we must be 'high functioning' and have little to no support needs.

Then there's the people who say that self-identifying isn't valid, that you can only be autistic if and when a doctor 'diagnoses' you. Yet many in our community can't access an assessment pathway – diagnosis is a privilege – and there are also many who choose to self-identify often after many years of self-exploration. We need to honour and embrace people's deep and intrinsic self-knowing. Those who self-identify are a part of the autistic community too – acceptance and belonging matters.

The invisible neuro minority

However we all got here, what we know is that historically our understanding of autism has been influenced and dominated by the male perspective, which has concealed the autistic experiences of women and those who are gender non-conforming. The stereotypical presentation of autism is male biased, with on average three times more boys than girls being diagnosed (Loomes *et al.*, 2017).

And although the prevalence of autism has been found *not to differ* across racial and ethnic groups, studies have found that 'White children and those of higher socioeconomic status are more likely to be both identified and diagnosed autistic earlier compared with Black and Brown children as well as children from low-income families' (Alyward *et al.*, 2021). These barriers and added intersectional layers of discrimination mean that many autistic women have gone undiscovered for many decades and, even at the point of late discovery, still have no choice but to self-identify. (Intersectionality in this context refers to being autistic and the overlapping nature of various different additional identities, such as race, gender, sexuality, class, and the interplay of those identities with autism, and how those intersectional identities further contribute to, and compound systemic oppression and discrimination.)

Added to this we know that 'despite efforts to increase the representation of autistic females in research, studies consistently enrol small samples of females or exclude females altogether' (D'Mello *et al.*, 2022). Consequently, our stories and our experiences go unheard and remain undiscovered, and we remain misunderstood.

We are the *invisible neuro minority* who were also invisible children – and even more invisible if we are black, brown, from a low-income family and/or gender non-conforming. We know through recent studies that gender diversity is more prevalent in the autistic community than the general population, and that sexuality appears to be more varied too (Kallitsounaki *et al.*, 2021) and that identifying as trans and autism frequently co-occur (Bouzy *et al.*, 2023).

And for all those who say that 'labels' don't matter, or that autism is 'only a small part of you' and not something you should 'define yourself by', I hope that this book gently challenges some of those misconceptions and beliefs, and shows why coming home to yourself is the route to self-acceptance and self-understanding and more compassionate awareness.

Late discovery

Late discovery is an area I'm hugely passionate about, and an area I hoped to focus my doctorate in psychology on. My Psychology Masters was supposed to be my springboard onto either the clinical or counselling doctorate here in the UK. However, despite putting myself through the ordeal of an interview, and being offered a place to study in London with the Metanoia institute, I had to have some real talk with myself and accept that doing my doctorate and having to travel to London from Yorkshire for four years was simply too much.

Pre-discovered me would have shamed myself into doing it, putting on a mask and pushing on through. Late discovered me knows the price I will pay to do that and it doesn't feel accessible. Rediscovered me says 'Hey, maybe try another, kinder way of doing this'. The Late Discovered Club was the solution.

I didn't need a doctorate; I was already *doing it*.

This for me was such an important area of work, yet I would have to self-fund my way through it because exploring the inner worlds of late discovered autistic women didn't seem to be any-one's research priority, and ultimately the decision to *not* do my doctorate came down to accessibility – both financially and phys-ically. Physically, I knew I wouldn't have the energy or the ability to regularly commute to London due to my health challenges, and nor would my young daughter cope with the separation anxiety that would create.

Having a disability, being a carer, and cost are all barriers that could be relatively easily overcome if the doctorate was offered online, or if they were funded, or had a scholarship available for actually autistic people who want to take up roles as clinical and counselling psychologists, so that we can better support autistic people in healthcare, and redirecting research budgets from being 'cure driven' to 'neuro-inclusive focused' – simple accommodations that would make such a difference to people like me.

Rather, I decided I would use my entrepreneurial, narrative psy-chology, creative and community building skills, partnered with my eldest daughter Caty's technical expertise, to create a podcast, a platform to shine a light on all these stories that have been excluded from the narrative. My drive was to be a role model for my own daughter, to deconstruct the stereotype, and give the next genera-tion visibility of autistic women.

I figured that this way I get to reach significantly more women and hear many, many more stories, and perhaps write a book (this book), instead of a doctoral thesis. One thing I knew for sure is that we needed to shine a light on those stories because every single autistic experience is a completely unique human experience – a kaleidoscope of colours and flavours. If you've met one human being you've met one human being, and that is no different for a human being who is autistic.

I wanted to discover the women who have had to navigate life behind a mask because our stories matter, your story matters, edu-cating people matters, changing the narrative matters, and I hoped that the podcast could do exactly that, and that these stories could become the lights of hope on someone else's dark runway.

And in creating that space with the podcast, community and my group peer support circles it not only gave late discovered autistic women a voice, *it gave me a voice*. For the first time in my life I spoke about my autistic self, unmasked, in the very first episode on the podcast that launched in December 2022. I aptly called it 'Be the Change' and it did indeed signal a huge transformational change in my life and my work.

A manifesto for change

In writing this book, interviewing the late discovered contributors and drawing on the most up-to-date research and studies *five clear themes* have emerged and these are themes that I want people to listen to, and act on, both for this present generation of autistic women, and the generations that come after. Throughout the book I will explore all of these themes in more depth.

1. Closing the health inequality gap

2. Being seen and heard

3. Access to neuro-inclusive assessments

4. Workplace inclusion

5. Support through the lifespan

Call it a manifesto for change.

Powering progress

Because we deserve to no longer be an invisible neuro minority of women.
 We deserve to be seen, heard, understood and supported.
 We matter.
 You matter.
 We deserve better, and future generations deserve better.

1. Closing the health inequality gap

These are the shocking truths that writing this book has uncovered for our community of late discovered autistic women. I can't find anywhere outside the pages of this book where these are presented in their entirety. The headlines are provided below and the detail and sources explored in more depth throughout the book.

Brace yourselves...

- We are 13 times more likely to die by suicide than women who aren't autistic and nine times more likely to experience suicidal ideation when compared with the general population (NHS England, 2023).

- We are more likely than non-autistic people to have chronic ill health, with diagnosed medical conditions across all nine organ systems and higher rates of 33 specific conditions compared to non-autistic people. This is also the first epidemiological study to show that Ehlers-Danlos Syndrome (EDS) may be more common among autistic women than non-autistic women (Ward *et al.*, 2023).

- We are more likely to experience polycystic ovarian syndrome, premenstrual tension, endometriosis, hypermobility, Ehler-Danlos Syndrome (EDS), epilepsy and myalgic encephalomyelitis/chronic fatigue syndrome (ME/CFS) as well as many other conditions (Ward *et al.*, 2023).

- We are more likely to experience co-occurring mental health conditions than non-autistic people. It is estimated that around a third of autistic people report a (diagnosed) mental health condition, whether this is more prevalent in autistic women is currently unknown (NHS England, 2023).

- We are more likely to be sexually victimized. We know that nine out of ten autistic women are sexually victimized, and that whilst sexual violence affects about 30 per cent of women in the general population it is between *two to three times* as much for autistic women. Being autistic means a 10–16 per cent risk of enduring sexual molestation as a child and a 62–70 per cent risk of being sexually victimized in adulthood; most victims are girls and women (Cazalis, 2022).

- We are more likely to be victims of interpersonal violence (Pearson *et al.*, 2022).

- We are more likely to experience potentially traumatic events (Haruvi-Lamdan *et al.*, 2020) and the *type* of trauma that we experience often doesn't look like the trauma that we see described in the DSM-5 (Happe *et al.*, 2020).

- We are more likely to experience problems with sleeping. In a recent study (Pavlopoulou & Dimitriou, 2018) over 70 per cent of autistic adults said they experienced difficulty falling asleep or staying asleep, associating this with sensory issues and high anxiety, and around half were unable to stay asleep for long, whilst four in ten experienced nightmares.

- We are more likely to experience autism-related difficulties (including sensory sensitivity, socializing with others, feeling suicidal and communicating needs) during the menopause (Moseley *et al.*, 2020).

- And underneath all of this, disparities in diagnosis remain. Female and Black populations are 'diagnosed later, are excluded from research as well as services designed for autistic people, and autistic black girls are effectively invisible in the current scientific literature'(Diemer & Regester, 2022).

Call to action

- We need social and relational support and guidance for autistic women and girls because we know that they are at a significantly higher risk of sexual victimization when compared to the general population and are more likely to experience interpersonal victimization – from parents, friends, colleagues and loved ones.

- We need relational advice and advocacy around coercive control, domestic abuse, support at the point of relationship breakdown, as well as navigating the divorce process that is tailored to our needs.

- We need more support in terms of suicide prevention – safety plans for when it is darkest should be a part of everyone's toolkit. We need spaces to speak out loud and hear others' experiences, as well as guidance to help ourselves understand our risks and triggers, and how we can reduce and mitigate them, not just for those who have been able to access a formal diagnosis but for all those women who self-identify.

- We need women's health specialists spanning both mental and physical health (whole body approach) who autistic women can be referred to with the knowledge and understanding of autism and co-occurring conditions to connect the dots and navigate and advocate the systemic challenges.

- We need GPs to understand the long list of co-occurring health and mental health conditions and the inner world experiences of autistic women, and to monitor our health care needs regularly, right through the lifespan as we hit menopause and beyond. We need them to believe us when we say we are in pain, and include our health stories as part of our autism assessment pathway.

- We need more scientific research and support services that centre the experiences of black and brown autistic women and girls, and those with additional intersectional identities and marginalized groups.

- We need therapists and mental health professionals in both private practice and across the NHS to better understand PTSD and co-occurring mental health conditions in autistic women and to use more neuro-affirming tools and adapted neuro-inclusive approaches to therapy.

- We need autism specific menopause support and interventions, and for our specific challenges and our vulnerabilities during menopause to suicide and mental health to be understood by our families, our communities and within the workplace.

There is very little to no research out there about autistic burnout in late discovered women and even less research about the psycho immunological connection between autistic burnout and chronic pain, illness, cancer and all the other ways that burnout wreaks havoc on our bodies – despite it being one of the universally collective experiences I have heard our community bond over – which means that there is little to no professional knowledge and technical 'know how' when it comes to assessment, treatment, prevention and recovery. We need to do more.

2. Being seen and heard

The Late Discovered Club Podcast isn't just storytelling, it's bringing narrative and a frame of reference to previously unheard and undiscovered autistic experiences of women and marginalized genders through an intersectional lens – experiences we need to hear and see more of.

The podcast is community led and is making a difference, and we want to continue bringing these hidden stories from invisible women and people. We've received so many reviews and messages from people whose lives this podcast is making a difference to which demonstrates how vital it is that we provide places and spaces for stories and experiences to be heard and shared.

'The Late Discovered Podcast! Oh my goodness I honestly can't articulate how helpful it has been for me. The number of times I've shouted "YES!" or finally understood why I do some things. Or realizing that actually some things I do most people don't. Many, many mind blowing moments.'

How do we know and learn about autism if our stories and our narrative have been missing from decades of being undiscovered and misunderstood? There is a need to ensure that our voices are being heard in our workplaces, in our health systems, in our communities, in schools and educational settings and in our homes too – especially those marginalized, intersectional voices, as one of our contributors explains below:

'Finding stories of other late discovered women in all shapes and forms: social media posts, articles, books, podcasts, real-life interactions, etc. especially non-white women and people with diverse SOGIESC [sexual orientations, gender identities and expressions]. It has been a bit difficult but whenever I come across stories from individuals from the global south, they have been the most useful treasures ever.'

Call to action

- We need more research which is led by the autistic community that also involves autistic women who self-identify – of whom there are many.

- We need to see and hear more stories from women who experience autism through an intersectional lens, right across the lifespan. These voices are missing and need to be heard and their experiences centred in the autistic experience.

- We need to identify the top research priorities for late discovered autistic women and direct funding to support and further explore the research priorities that matter most to late discovered women.

- We need funding to support more community led podcasts, projects and campaigns which centre late discovered autistic women's stories and experiences.

- We need a seat at the table whenever and wherever decisions are being made – nothing about us, without us.

3. Access to neuro-inclusive assessments

We know all too well in our Late Discovered Club Community that we experience multiple barriers to diagnosis, and that lived experience is underpinned by research which shows there is an increased recognition that autistic women face many barriers to formal diagnosis and are underserved by the clinical criteria and processes required to receive a diagnosis (Estrin *et al.*, 2020).

'We don't have the means for me to access a diagnosis privately. The first GP I spoke to was dismissive and asked me if I wanted a diagnosis because I was an influencer? (I'm not an influencer – I can't even influence my own toddler to eat his porridge.)'

'I'd had my lightbulb moment at that point but I didn't know what to do with it. I was in severe burnout, I couldn't get through a conversation without crying and just needed someone to show me some compassion and understanding. Instead, I was sent away with some Sertraline (which I've been prescribed on numerous occasions and never taken), a link to the NHS autism page and a sick note.'

'We need to be taken seriously and to have our struggles and trauma validated. The first time I went to the GP I was on my knees; my mental health was dead in the gutter and I didn't know where to turn or how to get myself together.'

Given that we know that these barriers exist, a more inclusive understanding of late discovered autism is needed. Self-identifying autistic women do exist and will too have support needs and mental health challenges. Their experiences are equally as valid as those autistic women, who against the odds, have received a formal diagnosis. Diagnosis saves lives; we also know through research (Davies *et al.*, 2024) that a positive autistic identity is associated with improved mental health and wellbeing.

Self-identifying often comes not through choice, but rather because of the multitude of barriers to accessing a diagnosis – not to mention the negative and stigmatizing perspective within many communities and families. Self-identifying is often the only option due to multiple (discriminatory) barriers that prevent access to a diagnosis pathway, and sometimes because there is no 'middle ground' between self-discovery and a formal diagnostic assessment.

'I do not feel the need to go through the NHS process. I looked into it and feel I am past that now. I would have liked to talk with professionals in the field about my revealings and journey onwards but I do not have the financial resources to continue to do so.'

'I wonder if in discovering our nature late in life we actually know ourselves more deeply and richly. I always thought that I was not the same as others, that I was in some way broken.

In recent years I felt I was ticking along through life in a low level of depression or only experiencing part of life. The revealing of my autistic nature washed all that aside. A massive flood of relief that I am ok. I am me. I just think differently. My brain works as it does. How it dives off down many avenues, becomes entangled and so noisy. The effect this had on my emotional and physical health.'

'In learning this and experiencing how to address my scrambled head I can have times of peace and clarity. I know what sends my brain off into overdrive and in this recognition I can pre-empt an overwhelm (not always!). But sometimes is good enough for me.'

Barriers to assessment is one of the areas we explore in The Late Discovered Club Podcast. Through these stories we can see how self-identifying for many brings a sense of self-knowing and self-understanding, after a lifetime of not knowing why you struggled. It's often after months and years of exploration and self-education.

In 2024 we polled our almost 8000-strong community on Instagram, of whom 95 per cent identify as women, and over a third of respondents self-identified as autistic.

Self-identifying is 100 per cent valid.

Your autistic identity is valid.

Call to action

- We need to educate the gatekeepers on autism in women and girls. I've heard far too many stories of professionals blocking referrals for assessments, or telling women and girls that they don't 'look autistic' and invalidating our own inner worlds and preventing women and girls from accessing the support they need to help frame their world.

- We need health professionals and workplaces to accept self-identification as valid to be able to access support, and to trust our own self-knowing.

- We need more affordable and timely access to neuro-inclusive, gender-specific assessments and options to assess parents/families at the point of child assessments.

- We need alternative options for those who do not want a formal diagnosis, but do want to explore their inner world and experiences with a professional who can facilitate that in a neuro-inclusive way.

4. Workplace inclusion

One of the many challenges that our late discovered autistic community faces is the need for more autistic-affirming and inclusive workplaces that feel safe places in which to self-disclose and create the safety anchors we need individually to prevent overwhelm, burnout and ill health.

This has featured in almost every single story I've explored on the podcast, because without psychologically safe workplaces, we mask and masking leads to burnout, and burnout affects our mental and physical health and wellbeing and we end up excluded and exiting out of workplaces because they *can't and won't* accommodate our individual needs.

There are a number of ways late discovered autistic women are discriminated against in the workplace which I explore in more depth in Chapter 11.

Added to this the UK Office for National Statistics (ONS, 2021) reported that only 22 per cent of autistic people were in work, the lowest among the disabilities they analysed, which means that autistic people still face the highest rates of unemployment of all disabled groups, and we experience many barriers in the workplace.

Call to action

- We need more neuro-affirming and autistic inclusive workplaces that feel like safe places in which to self-disclose and request adjustments. Women shouldn't feel that disclosure is a career limiting choice, and fear shouldn't be a barrier to seeking out adjustments.

- We need to get language right, and educate all staff on the neurodiversity paradigm.

- We need business leaders and shareholders within big corporations leading by example. The businesses that are incredibly profitable should be driving best practices.

- We need to work collaboratively with employers. We can achieve so much more together rather than as individuals.

- We need organizations to see the potential that autistic women can offer and then actively attract, recruit and retain autistic women employees through campaigns.

5. Support through the lifespan

Not only have we grown up firmly under the radar with that existential feeling of not belonging, when we do finally discover our autistic selves we find ourselves invalidated, dismissed and unsupported because we can't access the support that we need.

Without a doubt one of the biggest challenges our community faces is the feeling of isolation, loneliness and that sense that we don't belong (a common theme in our podcast stories). We've had a lifetime of it – which we know is what fuels the high rate of suicide amongst our population, and the high rate of mental health prevalence.

Furthermore, recent research tells us that 'peer support, and/or self directed support resources may be valuable mechanisms for supporting autistic people to cultivate a positive autistic identity' (Davies *et al.*, 2024).

We know that post discovery support circles are life changing and self-affirming – that's the feedback from the 150+ women who have taken part in the six-week online programme so far during 2022–2024. Women have participated from across the world, not just here in the UK.

We want to deliver more, both in person and online.

Call to action

- Over the next ten years we want to connect one million women and people through our circles, community and podcast and tailor support through the lifespan.

- We want to support women beyond menopause, through retirement and beyond, because late discovered autistic women who are elders, as well as those women who experience intersectional identities are especially invisible, and their needs are not understood, supported or accommodated in the places and spaces they find themselves in as a late discovered woman.

- We need more awareness and support, as well as a willingness to learn more, amongst health professionals, in the workplace and in our homes of the very real challenges we face across the lifespan.

One of our community contributors sums up what we need when it comes to support through the lifespan:

'We need more scientific research, greater awareness amongst GPs, nurses, mental health specialists, teachers, employers, parents, etc, earlier diagnosis, better support, guidance through the most challenging chapters (puberty, understanding relationships and friendships, motherhood, establishing ourselves in the workplace, work/life balance, wellbeing and emotional education).'

'All individuals need this, however autistic women are like the canaries in the coal mine – our sensitivity to these issues shines a light on the challenges they may present for many other people. These phases of transition are evidently more of a struggle for us (anxiety, depression, suicidal ideation, addictive behaviour, decimation of self-esteem) but everyone would benefit from more support according to their needs.'

'The DSM and the assessment process need to be better tailored to women. We need wider education in our communities about what the female experience of being autistic looks like. And we need to build better support for women diagnosed later in life who are managing not only our own needs, but those of our neurodivergent children.'

One of our community members talks about the impact of the loss of structure at the touch point of her retirement:

'I also think the structure I worked within provided a framework to hold my undiscovered and unrecognized autism. So being retired and a supposedly free agent in some ways I feel much more at sea.'

The five themes presented and explored in this chapter are important themes that we need people to listen to, and act on, both for this present generation of autistic women, and the generations that come after.

- Closing the health inequality gap

- Being seen and heard

- Access to neuro-inclusive assessments

- Workplace inclusion

- Support through the lifespan

As a late discovered community our needs and priorities aren't advocated for, nor are they represented or reflected in any large-scale research study, workplace initiative, or outlined in any government or health policy.

Whilst we may be a largely invisible neuro minority, we exist. Our needs matter.

And we deserve to be seen and understood and supported.

CHAPTER 3

Our Sensory World

There is no 'one way' of experiencing the world as an autistic person, and the 'how' is something that we experience uniquely and internally – what people 'see' are often the responses to sensory, emotional, cognitive and social overwhelm. There is no one who exists like you, which is why we need to give a voice to our individual experiences – we are not a monolith.

However, there are some common experiences that connect us together as a neuro minority of late discovered autistic women and people, and this chapter is going to explore that, along with helping you to understand you and how you perceive and react to the world around you, and identifying your sensory experiences.

Your power really lies in *you* understanding how *you* experience the world, and what that looks and feels like for you, and as we go through this chapter there are reflection points and experiences for you to draw on to help guide you on understanding this aspect of your autistic self, so that you feel empowered to self-advocate for your needs, and to seek out those adaptations and accommodations that will make the difference between you navigating your life in survival mode and thriving mode.

Our sensory world

Our sensory world is at the heart of how we experience the world, and our 'senses' – all eight of them – are the means by which our body perceives external stimuli. Our sensory system is rooted in human evolution and gives us the ability to understand, recognize and react to stimuli around us. However, for many autistic people, our senses can be over-responsive (hypersensitive), under-responsive (hyposensitive) or often a mix of both – and all very much context and environmentally dependent. The world can be a disabling place for autistic people.

There will be things that we seek to avoid and minimize because they cause us distress, rage, anger, irritability, frustration, overwhelm, stress, to feel repulsed, physically sick and/or pain and they can, and do, create disabling environments for us.

There are also things that we might seek out because of sensory input that we need – perhaps because something isn't registering on our sensory radar, or seeking out sensory joy, as well as the things we seek out to drown out or cancel out the things that feel too much, for example, replacing a triggering noise with a noise that feels soothing.

I like to think of it as having our own distinctive frequency that we need to tune into to feel regulated and to enable us to thrive, on an eternal daily quest to find that equilibrium we each need, and that looks different for each of us. In Chapter 12 you can find the 'Frequency Circle', which is a tool designed to place you at the centre of *your* own circle, tuning into your unique frequency, an alien concept when you've spent your entire life navigating a world that isn't accommodating for the way you experience it.

As autistic people, contrary to those who don't understand us and our neurology, continually exposing us to our sensory stressors does not mean that we eventually become desensitized or habituated to our sensory stressors. We instead from a very early age learn to mask, camouflage, assimilate and compensate, quickly learning that our responses to those sensory stressors in our environment are not acceptable in the neuronormative world in which we live – and just because others don't 'see' it, it doesn't mean we aren't experiencing it.

And *how* we experience the world can and does shift and change based on situations and variables. Stress, burnout, tiredness, pregnancy, pain, trauma, fluctuating hormones, menopause, illness, and the environments we find ourselves in, for example, can all impact on how we experience the world around us, often dialling up our sensory sensitivity or our need to seek out sensory input. Climbing the breast cancer mountain dialled all my sensory systems up high, as well as all the hormonal changes from crashing into a chemo-induced menopause – I'm having to continually readjust my frequency to meet myself where I find myself at.

The key bit here is to understand *you* and *your* sensory world.

What that looks like and feels like for *you.*

Working out the things, the external sensory stressors that dial up your senses or dial them down.

Where and how you find your calm and peace in a world that feels too much.

Allowing ourselves to unpack our sensory worlds, without the tyranny of the 'should' or sitting under the veil of shame or the heavy weight of invalidation, but with a sense of curiosity and inquisitiveness, self-observation, openness and compassion.

Ask yourself 'what do I need?'

What are some of the signs that you need to pay more attention to?

What aspects of your needs have you suppressed and been gaslighted into invalidating?

What would change if you gave yourself permission to advocate for yourself and to prioritize your needs?

And one of the biggest challenges in our late discovery is the unravelling.

Rediscovering ourselves means that we begin to unpack and unravel decades of sensory trauma which has been enforced through social expectations and external invalidation. The realization that our sensory needs were ridiculed, punished, pushed down, eye rolled, and what is so often the case, never met, but suppressed because we never had the lens or the narrative in which to frame our needs, and our needs were seen as being 'too much' or that we are 'too sensitive' or too 'dramatic'.

It's no wonder so many late discovered autistic women and people hit burnout and experience poor mental and chronic ill health.

Neither is it any surprise that the body screams enough so frequently and so loudly when our nervous system has spent decades in a place of dysregulation and we've had to mask our way through life to exist in a world that really isn't built for or accommodating of our needs.

'I've been really lucky – I moved to Dubai when I was in my 20s and here there is no "normal". It's a very multicultural, multinational place, so some of my Quirks are much less obvious than they would be in a more homogeneous society like the UK.'

'I can use cultural norms here like modesty as part of my armour – I don't have to touch or be touched as much. I can avoid loud places and stick in the quieter female spaces. I think it's made a big part of me functioning as well as I have over the years.'

Our sensory system

Our sensory experiences impact how we interact with others and with the world around us. When we think of our senses, we may think of the most obvious ones – *taste, smell, touch, visual and sound;* however, there are also three additional, less talked about senses that also matter in terms of how we as humans experience the world from a sensory perspective, and these three senses are prominent in the autistic sensory experience.

Proprioception

Proprioception is the sense of awareness of our own body; it communicates data to us about how our body parts are moving. If we are under-responsive, we are likely going to seek out the sensory input that we need, which might look like biting/chewing, hyper extending joints, deep pressure such as tight bear hugs, or a weighted blanket, weight bearing and cardio.

Conversely, hypersensitivity can make it difficult to understand where your body is in relation to other objects which might look like knocking things over or having difficulty in regulating pressure with objects.

Interoception

Whilst interoception may be less well known than our other senses, we are learning more and more about how our sensitivity to interoceptive signals can determine our capacity to regulate our emotions, and the subsequent impact on our mental health.

Interoception helps us to form our most basic sense of self, and our interoceptive awareness is our internal sense of how we experience and regulate what's going on in our body – everything from temperature, pain, to hunger and thirst, and it's our interoceptors (our internal sensors) that let us know what our internal organs are feeling. We can over-respond to some types of pain, yet under-respond to other types of pain, and the same goes for medication too.

A recent study (Trevisan *et al.*, 2021) explored the firsthand accounts of adults who self-identify as autistic describing their interoceptive challenges. Many described 'limited awareness of hunger, satiation, or thirst. Others described limited awareness or difficulty understanding affective arousal, pain or illness, and difficulty differentiating benign body signals from signals that represent medical concerns.' The study called for increased research attention on this topic.

Interoception, it seems, is one of our most important senses, and therefore if we struggle to register it, or we register too much of it, there's no wonder that it causes us such overwhelm and impacts on our mental health and wellbeing. Which means finding ways of understanding our interoceptive needs, and importantly, ways of tuning into ourselves is an important part of our own rediscovery.

Vestibular

Our vestibular system tells us where our body is in relation to gravity, where it is moving to, and how fast. If we are over-responsive to vestibular input we may struggle with motion sickness – think travel sickness, elevators and escalators which can be debilitating – and if we are under-responsive we are going to need to seek out sensory experiences to stimulate our vestibular sense, which can look like a need to be on the go all the time – swings, rides, dance – anything that stimulates our movement and balance.

Synaesthesia

This is where an experience we have comes in through one sensory system and goes out through a different sensory system. This can look and feel like, for example, hearing a sound but experiencing it as a colour, or seeing shapes as emotions, or perceiving tastes when looking at words and certain sounds can induce sensations in the body.

My sensory experiences

Pre-discovery I was oblivious to how and why I experienced the world on a sensory level, until I hit a point where I could no longer mask the pain and discomfort. Part of my own rediscovery journey was to allow myself to be an observer in my own world, to be curious about what my sensory world looked like, of how those sensory triggers made me feel, and what dialled up my sensory perceptions, as well as what helped to regulate them.

What was my sensory frequency and what *disrupted* and *moderated* that frequency?

As I began to be sensory curious and open to sensory exploration, I dug deep into my past experiences but also allowed myself to be aware of what was happening in the present on a day-to-day basis for me. I took pictures of sensory triggers and built up a sensory photo album on my phone, and when I couldn't take pictures of an experience, I wrote it down in my notebook and eventually developed a spider diagram, not just of my sensory triggers, but of my response – the thoughts, the feelings (which I found hard to identify), the behaviours, and the physical feelings in my body that followed.

Movement has always been something that I have sought out – running, swimming, trampolining, high jumping, long jumping, tap dancing, and the thrill of a rollercoaster. As I looked backwards, I discovered that many of my childhood memories related to sensory trauma, with food featuring prominently.

Taste

Food for me has always been an issue, and it's a common shared experience in our late discovered community too.

> 'More of an issue is the texture of foods – it took me years to eat eggplant – the skin of it was unnaturally squeaky – like a dolphin. There's no way you could make me eat cottage cheese or fish. The smell and texture just mean I couldn't get the fork to my mouth ever.'

I have vivid memories of eating meat as a child and being physically sick by the texture and the taste of it, and of hiding food that made me feel sick from my plate, in my pockets under the dinner table. I have aversions to many foods because of how they look, smell, taste and how they make me feel, which has meant a restrictive and limiting diet. I live off 'safe' foods and find myself in cycles of eating the same food on repeat until I eventually can't eat it any longer and have to find a new 'safe' food.

I can't eat seafood, most fish and meat, and often eggs because of the smells and textures, and I feel a visceral aversion when it comes to eating anything that comes from a living animal and the connection my mind makes to another living being, especially when I don't know where it has come from, or the kind of life it has lived before it ends up on my plate. If I allow myself to think about it I feel repulsed.

During my chemotherapy treatment my body was craving meat (especially red meat) despite the fact I have avoided meat for a significant number of years. The urge to eat it was so overpowering, and during that period of treatment where all my cells were being obliterated – both healthy ones and cancerous ones – it felt as though my body dialled down my sensory system for me, just enough to enable me to get the nutrients it needed for cell renewal and healing from such a toxic treatment. I switched to plant milk about 20 years ago, yet during my pregnancy my body craved cows' milk and I drank it in pint loads – it seems that when my body knows what it needs it will do whatever it needs to alert me to that fact.

I am rule driven when it comes to food. If I or somebody presents rules when it comes to food I can stick to them with relative ease. Eating out brings a whole lot of anxiety with it, and I will always opt for the 'safest' food on the menu which will do the least amount of triggering my hypersensitive gut. Going on holiday I have to quickly establish myself in a new routine of food, and once I find something that works, fits and doesn't cause me to be ill I will stick to it for the foreseeable.

My eating habits are not driven by a desire to lose weight. They are driven by rules and by safety, of knowing that the food I put in my mouth will not cause me to be sick because of the taste, smell or texture, or cause me gastrointestinal issues. Even 'safe' foods can cause me distress, especially fruit, the rogue strawberry that is too soft, the apple that isn't crisp enough or the orange that isn't quite juicy enough.

I feel disgust when different textures of foods touch each other – eggs and avocado for me are a big no – and I'm disappointed when I reach the boredom stage with my 'safe' foods because I've been eating them on repeat.

I have rules around the order I need to eat my food in and how it's presented. The crockery I use and the cups and glasses for different types of drinks matter. The feeling of food in my body, and how it makes me feel dictates how I eat – I don't like the physical feeling of fullness.

I have had emotional meltdowns over food as an adult, fuelled when I have been focused on what I'm going to eat only to discover that it's already been eaten, and have also found myself ridiculed for what must look, from the outside, like a very controlling and limiting way to navigate food. Through an autistic lens I can now see why, and through a self-compassionate lens I can understand why it matters to me and to give myself the permission to eat in a sensory friendly way (for me).

I'm not failing as a human being because I want to eat the same safe foods on repeat every day. I can and do recognize how and why my approach to food would be labelled as 'avoidant' and 'restrictive' (ARFID); however for me, it's a work around I have found that pacifies my sensory system, and tunes into my sensory frequency.

ARFID stands for Avoidant Restrictive Food Intake Disorder and is characterized by avoiding foods or types of foods which leads to a restrictive way of eating. ARFID can be experienced for several reasons including sensory issues, gastrointestinal problems, distressing experiences with food, a lack of appetite, mealtime environments which might be overwhelming and/or anxiety inducing, or difficulty with interoception which might mean missing the internal signal that we are hungry.

It can show up as:

- anxiety around getting stomach pain/IBS type symptoms from food or being sick

- avoiding eating or trying foods due to the smell, texture, taste, or how they look

- only eating foods in a certain way, order or temperature

- having a limited or narrow amount of food groups

- feeling anxious during mealtimes

- needing to eat alone due to the overwhelm of the environment

- having 'safe' foods and eating on repeat

- needing to know in advance what's on the menu/meal planning.

Current research recognizes that autism is seen in those with ARFID at higher rates than the general population rate of 1.5 per cent.

Estimates of co-occurring ARFID and autism range from 12.5 per cent all the way up to 33.3 per cent (Harris *et al.*, 2019, Inouye *et al.*, 2021). But as with any of these studies, they don't take into account the late discovered community and food is a hot topic within our community. Our experiences have so far gone under the radar and have been largely undiscovered.

Sound

Noise and sound is a big sensory trigger for me and many in our community. But it's also a sensory soother in that the right sounds, delivered in the right way, attuned to my frequency can also be soothing and self-regulating, namely fire, nature, soothing jazz, smooth music, water and calming voices.

> 'Certain sounds can dysregulate me in a second, and trigger a sensation of white-hot fury and panic. Loud motorbikes revving, yapping dogs, vehicles hooting, pneumatic drills, people shouting, kids screaming – any sudden blast of sound makes me jump out of my skin. However, music is a source of profound autistic joy for me.'

I need complete quiet and calm to sleep, and to work, which is why in my old work life of world travel, overnight hotel stays and open plan offices had such an impact on my nervous system, and why I need autonomy over the where and how to make it a more sensory friendly experience.

I listen to the same songs on repeat, having curated a soothing playlist that I listen to whilst 'doing' – either whilst driving or when I'm cooking. I get overwhelmed by voices, spaces and noises that are loud, sudden and when there are multiple noises layered together, or if someone is talking to me whilst I'm doing something else. I very quickly lose my concentration, my ability to speak, and it hurts my head, it feels like the frequency becomes muddled and screechy.

'I struggle with layers of noise – if the extractor fan is on in the kitchen and the TV is on or someone is trying to talk to me I can't deal with it. Also, if someone tries to talk to me over the TV or music in general. I actually feel rage! It's taking me a while to find them all, but now that I'm in a calmer state and my nervous system has recovered somewhat I'm noticing what puts me on edge. It's a steep learning curve!'

Noise can become magnified and if I'm at the hairdressers, at the hospital, on a train, in the school playground at pick up, or a cafe or restaurant or somewhere with lots of sounds and multiple conversations happening all at the same time, I find it exhausting to have to endure, and need ample downtime to decompress and retune into my frequency to feel regulated.

Now I understand the rediscovered version of me, I know that I can make the adaptations I need, and ask for accommodations, for example, the quietest table in the restaurant, or headphones and/or my loop earplugs in at the hairdressers and on the train, a quieter room to wait in at the hospital. In the past, I must have found a way of zoning out and somehow enduring the dysregulation – but for whom, and to what detriment?

I'm grateful that I had this discovery pre breast cancer treatment, and that I was able to put narrative to my experiences in hospital and to understand *why* the hospital environment, particularly on unplanned, acute hospital stays triggered meltdowns. Too much noise, and too many different types of noise, layered on top of pain engulfed my nervous system. My knowledge meant that I could advocate for myself, make the adaptations I needed and seek out the accommodations that would help calm my nervous system, although they haven't always been heard, understood or accommodated by others during my treatment and hospital stays.

And I discovered that sound baths, breathwork and sound meditation are next level sensory soothers and where I find joy. They speak to my frequency and instantly tune me in, dialling up my relaxation response, or what others might call 'rest and digest' something I will go into more depth over in Chapter 12 in my 'Frequency Circle' – a tool designed to help you put yourself at the centre of your own circle.

Smells

I have an aversion to many smells, especially the smell of certain foods and the smell of cooking certain foods, and I can 'smell' people, places and their scents which can be overpowering. Animal smells, body odour and uncleanliness make me feel disgust.

I've worn the same Chanel perfume for over a decade, and stick to the same familiar smells when it comes to personal hygiene products. I find incense and many scented candles too much, but once I find a scent I can tolerate I will buy on repeat, and I love the smell of fresh coffee and freshly cut grass.

'I can have physical reactions to smells, especially if they are unpleasant. Smells connected to specific foods and, more importantly, those that are connected to human bodies are truly the worst triggers for me.'

'This makes navigating crowded spaces even more uncomfortable, such as public transportation whereby close interaction with other people is unavoidable. If any of those people around me has an unpleasant smell, it will make the entire experience unbearable for me.'

During chemotherapy, my smell sensitivity became even more heightened to the point that even the 'safe' scents that I can normally tolerate became too much. I could smell the chemical scent of chemo on my skin which was intoxicating, yet nobody else could smell me.

Undergoing chemotherapy treatment for cancer, I experienced just about every single side effect that was listed. Days after my first chemotherapy cycle I became seriously ill and, despite lowering subsequent doses, each cycle the cumulative effects meant my whole body suffered the brutality of chemotherapy. I have always had a sensitivity to medication and I feel pain intensely, so it's no wonder then that chemotherapy affected me the way it did.

Despite receiving my treatment at one of Europe's largest cancer centres here in the UK, there was very little to no knowledge amongst my oncology team about the relationship between autism and chemotherapy and zero research that I could find.

However, my consultant radiologist totally got the relationship between autism and radiotherapy and how if I feel the world more intensely and sensitively that it's likely I will feel the effects of radiation being blasted into my body more intensely too. It's also encouraging to hear that the charity Breast Cancer Now has announced in 2023 funded research into the autistic experience of breast cancer and treatment to help further our understanding.

Touch

I never really appreciated how much I need touch to feel regulated, but equally I am sensitive to 'what' and 'how' touches my body. It's always a topic of conversation in our community too, especially within the context of navigating family and day-to-day life.

'I hate a lot of the touch sensations that my kids like which is challenging – I can't abide fleece or plushies, which are in my face a lot. If they touch me, it's like they instantly suck the moisture out of my body.'

'My kids always told me that I have not been very good at showing emotions, hugging etc – they'd always even ask to see my friend up the road because she gave them "nice hugs" – of course I did, and do hug my kids, but I have to really be intentional about it as I find touch really challenging sensory wise, so now with a diagnosis the kids and my husband are able to understand more and not take it as a personal thing.'

Deep massage, sensual touch, bear hugs, feeling cocooned under my duvet – these are things that I seek out. However, I'm also hyper-sensitive when it comes to what I wear and what I sleep on. The softer and least restrictive the better is my motto; if I feel restricted in what I'm wearing I very quickly begin to feel dysregulated. If it has a zip or doesn't come with an elasticated waist I will no longer wear it. I wear the same underwear, bra and socks from the same shop, and tights are a sensory nightmare if they are not 'just right'. I live for winter and the ability to cover every inch of my body in comforting clothes – hats and scarves are my thing.

My preference would be to live in a country that was cold all year round, that would be the ultimate in tuning into my frequency. I now understand why I'm drawn to the ice kingdoms of the north and why I like to visit Scandi countries in the depths of winter, and why the idea of a summer escape doesn't really appeal, and feeling too hot in my clothes is enough to push me over the edge. I'm forever in search of the 'just right' temperature.

The freedom of working for myself over the last decade has meant that I no longer have to wear clothes that are prescribed; I can dress how I *need* to dress, not how I'm *expected* to dress. I'm not sure how I managed at school and in the world of work, but do now have an appreciation of how dysregulated my nervous system must have been.

I can't swim in the sea or any open water because the thought of anything touching my skin makes me feel physically sick. I joined my local triathlon club when I could no longer run for the swimming and cycling part and the only way I could get in the water in my local reservoir was to be covered head, hands and toe in a wetsuit, gloves, hat, goggles, earplugs and close my eyes under the water so I couldn't see. I needed complete sensory deprivation to swim.

My open water swimming days didn't last long, and I couldn't work out why I couldn't do what others were doing? I love being outdoors and in nature but beach holidays and open water swimming are no longer part of my frequency, and that's ok.

Visual

Our eyes are the windows to our soul, and the visual windows through which we see and receive the world. For me too much visual stimuli quickly results in overwhelm.

> 'So much information comes in through my eyes and I now realize I have adopted a kind of tunnel vision to dampen this. When I go into any environment I am subconsciously aware and very vigilant of what is going on (visual, movement, auditory) and can work out a starting point of where to enter the situation.'

I talked in Chapter 1 about eye contact and the visual overwhelm I experience, and I now know why my sunglasses are a visual aid for me because the sunlight hurts my eyes. But it's more than that, I also feel protected when I wear them, an extra layer removed from what my eyes are constantly consuming, and I also now know why working online delivering training and therapy feels less intrusive than in person.

It was because of the pandemic in 2020 that I pivoted to online delivery, *not* the outcome of an adaptation I made to accommodate myself, and I very quickly discovered that working on a screen from an environment I have control over, without the daily assault of a commute, was tuning into my frequency. Because on a screen I don't have to look at anyone's eyes, I'm looking at my camera and I can minimize the room and choose a soothing background image.

Visually, I need my environment to be clutter free and less really is more. I enjoy the simplicity, clean lines, the minimalism and calmness of Scandi design, but equally I love colour and dressing happy with colour, experimenting with colour combinations – but the colour has to flow. From what I wear, to the environments I'm in, my sensory frequency is monochromatic.

I went forest bathing for my 44th birthday with a group of friends and I hadn't ever noticed how monochromatic the colour of the forest is, until our forest guide invited us to look up and experience it.

What I noticed was how it made me feel – the various shades of green had such a calming effect on my nervous system, and that's how I dress too. I pick a colour and will wear varying shades of that colour, or a combination of colours that flow.

Being attuned to my sensory frequency, making the adaptations I need and seeking out the accommodations that will help – for me, this is self-compassion in action. But to do that, we have to understand ourselves, and we have to be accepting of that rediscovered version of ourselves that we are becoming, and to show ourselves the grace and compassion that we so freely show others.

My world may have become smaller in many ways as a result of my rediscovery and climbing the breast cancer mountain along with chronic pain and physical ill health, but it has undoubtedly become deeper, richer, more authentic and significantly calmer, and it can only grow outwards from here when there is self-knowing and self-acceptance at its core.

I'm accepting of what my world needs to look like for me, and at peace with the idea that it might not look 'typical' from the outside looking in. I often look back in disbelief about how I managed to live my life the way I used to, before 'coming home'. I am mindful of the long-term health effects on my body from living in a world that really isn't built for my neurotype, and how much suffering I have endured.

Coming home is a feeling like no other, and I want you to be able to experience that feeling too.

 ## UNDERSTANDING *YOUR* SENSORY EXPERIENCES

In your rediscovery journey, this is a starting point for you to begin to be more observant of how you interact with the world on a sensory level. When I explored my own sensory world I imagined I was an anthropologist, immersed in my own world, but detached and separate enough from it to be able to watch, witness and distinguish some greater understanding of what my sensory needs are.

The anthropologist in me was systematic in my approach, with eight sensory domains to theme my observations around.

The outcome of the study I was undertaking was to understand how I experienced the world on a sensorial level and what needed to change in my world so that I could be more accommodating of my needs.

As part of your rediscovery I invite you to become the anthropologist sent on a mission to observe your sensory world. Not only are you going to immerse yourself in your own world, consider interviewing participants – parents, loved ones, friends, siblings – to gain some understanding of what they see and observe.

- What do you notice about your sensory triggers and needs? In seeking out and sensitivity? What dials it up or down?

- What can you learn about past experiences, and what are you observing in the present?

- What does it feel like when you experience a sensory trigger? For example, do you feel stressed, angry, frustrated, pain, discomfort?

  - How and where does it show up in your body?

  - How do you react? For example, do you cry, fight, flight, freeze, become angry or shut down?

- What do you notice are some of the signs that you need to pay more attention to? What aspects of your needs have you suppressed and why?

And an important question to ask and explore is what brings you sensory joy? What are the joy seeking experiences you seek out? What are your sensory soothers that help soothe your nervous system? And what are your sensory connectors and modulators, what helps connect you and what helps to modulate your sensory and nervous system?

Sensory soothers are anything for you that comes to your rescue during times of distress, when your sensory system has become overwhelmed. Sensory modulators are the everyday things you do to help you modulate your sensory system. Sensory connectors are the things that help you connect deeply to your senses.

Now that you have collated this research from your study about your sensory needs, what can you now identify that you need to change within your world? As you write up your research what would your recommendations be? Imagine giving yourself the permission to advocate for yourself and to prioritize your needs?

- What adaptations can you make (the things that sit within your control) and what accommodations can you seek out (the things that sit outside your control)?

- What do you need to do more of/less of?

- What do you need to give yourself permission to do?

This may be an exercise that you keep coming back to; for me it was a two-year work in progress. But what I found by becoming the anthropologist and the observer of my own world was that the more I took myself out of my own head and into the role of observer, the more I noticed, and the more I noticed the more aware I became, and the more aware I became the more I felt attuned to my body, and the more attuned I became the more I was able to advocate for myself and make changes that I needed.

And once I'd watched, witnessed and distinguished all of that, there was no going back to the undiscovered world with that view out of the steamed-up window.

- What do you really need to 'come home' to yourself?

CHAPTER 4

Our Emotional World

This chapter focuses on our emotional world, and what that can look and feel like when you are autistic. One of the standout discoveries on my own journey was the stark realization that I express and process my emotions differently from the neuro norm.

But that doesn't mean I don't feel them, because I do – I feel them deeply and pictorially and I'm a sponge for other people's energy and emotions too. I feel other people's pain – you might say that I'm hyper-empathetic, my empathy thermostat is dialled up high, which is why the world often feels a lot.

For as long as I can remember I have spent a lot of time in my own head, processing, analysing, making sense of what I'm feeling and why I'm feeling it (after the event, however, not in the event), which others around me have described as being 'deep, intense and serious'. I've studied human behaviour and how our minds work through to Master's level over a 20+-year period, read voraciously on the subject, and dedicated my career over the last decade to helping people understand themselves too.

'I would say that the way in which I experience the world is very intense, both physically, psychologically and emotionally. Everything I see or hear has meaning for me, and this can make the world seem beautiful one moment and very dark the next.'

I can take in big emotions, withstand other people's traumas, bear witness to their stories, and I'm immoderately calm in a crisis. Over the last decade as a therapist I've easily spent more than 10,000 hours inside the minds of others doing exactly that. I have a huge storage space that I've rented out in my head for other people's emotions, yet it feels like I have a mere matchbox for mine – an imbalance I have taken action to address in my rediscovered world.

In my own emotional world, my delayed processing of emotions, and a difference in outwardly expressing those emotions might be perceived by others as being emotion *less*, when in actual fact I'm emotion *full* because I feel things so very deeply and in abundance. I feel so much, all the time, and I'm all too aware of the need to make sense of *what* I'm thinking and *why* I'm feeling. I can't 'just' feel something. I have to understand 'why' I'm feeling it, dissect it, and I have to make sense of it in order to process it. It's a processing difference, not a deficit or something I lack.

I recognize that I sense-make by applying my inner experiences and emotions to something I can explain through a visual metaphorical picture in my mind – a mountain, a submarine, an earthquake, being at sea without an anchor, a matchbox, a brave new world are just a few of the sense-making visuals my mind has created and talked about so far in this book to help you the reader to hopefully try and understand my inside world, and it stands out to me that this depth, this ability that my beautiful autistic mind has to absorb, deep dive and sense make brings meaning to our collective human experience.

During one of the most traumatic and turbulent years of my life, I created and then drew the image of being inside the destructive force of a tornado, things happening around me and me being in the middle trying my hardest to stand my ground and not fall over, and then finding myself on a tightrope between two mountain tops trying my hardest not to fall off. Reading that back now, in hindsight, I can see through the pictures I created how traumatizing and scary that time was, yet on the outside looking in, nobody would have known.

And in contrast I've created visual places I go to in my mind, or will visit those places when I need to feel grounded and held, which are by default always nature connected. In my rediscovered world, rocks and big sturdy trees remind me of my strength. They have weathered storms and represent stability and resilience. They are full of energy and ageless wisdom and the way that they adapt in the face of adversity makes me stand in awe and admiration and I imagine that they are reflecting that back at me. That 'feeling' the rocks and trees embody in me is one of strength.

My mind wants and needs to tell a story with pictures to be able to say what and how I'm feeling, and that takes time to create. More recently, through an autistic dance project I've been collaborating with, I've been experimenting with translating those pictures into movement, and what I realized in my rediscovery is that I actually have a very elaborate toolbox that helps me to process my emotional world, and that I'm always adding to it.

My emotional processing might *look* different, but it's got depth and meaning and I understand it now, and I can appreciate how creative it is and how I've harnessed it in my work, and the transformative impact my brain, my neurotype, has had in a significant number of people's stories, and indeed my own story. In my rediscovered world I can see it for the immense strength that it actually is, but I can also honour and acknowledge my struggles and how disabling the world can be when you process the world so deeply and intensely and the places that I can go to when the world feels too much – something I explore in more depth in Chapter 6.

Inside and outside

It was during the pandemic, and the shift from in-person to online working on Zoom that I noticed, in ample disbelief, my facial expressions and emotional responses don't match my inner experiences. There is a clear mismatch from what I'm feeling on the inside and what I'm displaying on the outside. This discovery mortified me at the time because I got a glimpse of what others must see, and perhaps some insights into people's perceptions of me.

It takes real effort for me to show through my facial expressions and my body language what I'm feeling, especially joy and happiness. My facial expressions are largely monotone, and if I'm having a photo taken I have a 'go to' smile which isn't at all natural – it actually feels distressingly unnatural. I instead express myself and convey my emotions through the tone of my voice, my energy, my touch, my written word, and eventually when there is too much emotion I can no longer contain internally, it comes gushing out in the form of a tsunami of tears, what I term my 'overspill'.

'I am a very emotional person. I cannot stop my emotions. I have had people in the past tell me not to cry or to stop crying but I can't just stop. I feel my emotions in my body, especially in my chest and heart. Also in my gut. I feel my emotions very physically.'

I am super attuned to other people's facial expressions, energy, body language and tone of voice, and will 'read the room' with the nuances behind the outward facing behaviours they display, distinguishing subtle cues that others don't see or pick up on, quickly establishing whether there's a safety anchor there. I can feel the emotional dismissal and lack of safety hit me hard; however, when I allow myself to be sensitive to my experiences, I can now recognize and see that it's the layers of cumulative trauma that sit under numerous situations where people are covertly dismissive, uninterested and unkind.

Creating emotional safety isn't just in what people say, it's how they say it, it's in their tone of voice, it's in their body language, it's in their energy, and I'm here for the people who give me safety anchor vibes, but others interpret it as me being overly sensitive to situations. What they don't see from the outside looking in are the experiences I've had throughout my life.

When I did the reflecting back part of my rediscovery I remember not having any *immediate* or expected outward emotional response to my parents getting divorced when I was nine, or family members who passed away during my teens and early adulthood. I recognize that when it comes to grief and sadness I banish it inside one of my matchboxes to my emotional submarine, lock it away behind the airtight door until I'm ready to confront the torrent of emotion I know will come – perhaps it's a safety mechanism to protect me from inner overwhelm and the pain that comes with feeling emotion so deeply. Just as I order and compartmentalize all aspects of my day-to-day conscious living life, I also do this with emotionally charged experiences. I process them when I'm ready to withstand them.

On the outside looking in, it looks like I go through life without struggle, that I am somehow superhuman, the crisis handler equipped with this immense storage space open 24/7 for others to fill. Always 'fine' and always together. It means never really been seen, being wholly misunderstood, and bearing the weight of stacked up cumulative emotion.

Part of my own rediscovery has been identifying and understanding what I *need*, and working out the ways that help me to process and express my emotions. Ultimately I've concluded that I need to create more space for me, a more expansive space, with room to explore and express myself safely and in the ways that I know work for me – giving notice on the matchbox that has been my inner sanctum for the last four-and-a-bit decades.

Compassionate awareness

I recently discovered somatic flow yoga on a 'Profound Rest' retreat which involved three days of complete silence, a retreat I attended two months after my radiotherapy treatment and the first time on my mountain climb that I had actually stopped, taken off my walking boots and been whisked off to a healing sanctuary on the mountainside with space to confront for the first time what I had been through so far and how hard and high I had climbed. Whether it was the inner stillness of the silence, the invitation of embodied healing through the release of stuck emotions, or the visualization of my lungs letting go of grief and trauma through each and every breath, what flowed for me in that very first session were tears. Big, fat, wet tears engulfed me and I couldn't and didn't want to make them stop.

I was compassionately aware of the pain my body was in – every part from my fingertips to my feet, my knees and elbows, my hips and back were loudly letting me know that I needed to turn my attention to the pain, to invite it in and to sit with it and listen to it. And whilst I struggled to move my body beyond the basics, it was the sense of flow and somatic embodiment that was the magic ingredient here, combined with the compassionate awareness.

We were invited by Paris Ackrill, the guide and co-founder of The Broughton Sanctuary here in Yorkshire, to imagine that we are the loving mother holding our baby in my arms, lovingly and intuitively tending to her needs – only we are both the mother *and* the baby. That was such a powerful and transformative image for me to embody.

Breathing in and out through my lungs, letting go of sadness and grief, letting in compassionate awareness. Moving with my body and allowing my body to lead, soothing myself and letting go of the pain through tears. This was me embodying my emotions and I learned a lesson about compassionate awareness.

- For me it's about being aware of the pain I'm in.

- Allowing myself the aids I need to assist with that pain.

- Giving myself permission to move somatically in the way my body needs, even if that looks different to everyone else.

- It's not being critical or judgemental.

- It's acknowledging what my body has endured.

- It's letting go of the (more able) version of me that once was.

- It's letting in the current version of me.

- It's letting go of the shame I feel for my body not working the way it does for others.

- It's meeting myself where I am at.

- It's honouring my pain and holding curiosity for what could or might be different in the future.

This was another lesson for me in my emotional processing, a signal that to liberate those stuck emotions I need to add input and that flowing tears are not to be avoided. Tears are my emotional release, they serve a therapeutic role, and my sensitivity is an intrinsic part of who I am.

I know now that my body needs signals and input, in addition to a safe space, place and/or face, to process and express my emotions – my curated playlist of deep and meaningful songs in the car, watching emotive films, expressive writing, journaling, crying, drawing, group peer support, researching to make sense of something, space and solitude, sound meditation, somatic movement, kirtan (which is another form of meditation but one that involves singing to mantras), sound baths, running (pre hip and back problems) and swimming are the tried and tested ways that I have sought out ways to process and express my emotions.

> 'Journaling helps profoundly with processing my emotions. It gives me the time to express what I've been suppressing. It allows me to process what I'm feeling in the depth that I need and at my own pace.'

Pre-discovery I couldn't formulate why I found talking therapy on the other side of the couch as the client so painfully arduous. I now know that it's because the 'on demand' nature of talking therapy is not conducive to my flavour of emotional processing and expression. Add in the therapists who are oblivious to the need to adapt their way of working, and have zero knowledge and understanding about how the autistic neurotype works, or the cumulative trauma they don't recognize or see that so often shows up as PTSD and it's no wonder so many other autistic people struggle with unadapted, non-neuro-inclusive talking therapy, and then disengage and struggle with their mental health, hitting crisis point after crisis point, and then medication or in-patient care is the only solution on offer.

However, therapy that is adapted, affirming of our neurotype and feels safe can be, and is, life-saving for autistic people, and I know this because I've seen it in action with my own therapy clients. Creating neuro-inclusive spaces and neuro-inclusive practice in the therapy room for autistic people is something I'm extremely passionate about – I've guest lectured on this very subject at UCL, contributed to a book on the subject and co-authored a framework on what neuro-inclusion looks like in terms of space and approach in therapy.

'I struggle most with the fact that my emotional reactions are often much larger than those of people around me, and I can come across as very teary due to over-empathy or as very angry due to a heightened sense of justice.'

'Talking through my emotions is what helps me to process and recognize them. This can be in the context of therapy or with a friend or my partner. It can even be by myself in my head. I often write them down in the notes on my phone too. I always try to come up with a list of reasons that I am feeling the way that I am, so as to make sense of my emotions.'

'Reading books and listening to music also helps me. I can find myself empathizing very deeply with a character or their experience and realize I have had a similar emotional experience. When I feel overwhelmed either with joy or sadness I have playlists which will evoke those emotions and enable me to stim and dance or to cry the feelings through/out.'

My meditation practice is largely where I have processed my grief and trauma. For many of my sessions during this period of rediscovery I would emerge with tears streaming down my face; it felt like taking a pumice stone to a lifetime of 'stuck' and unprocessed grief and emotion, with each session of my practice clearing the backlog. The body does indeed 'keep the score', and my body is no exception.

Through reading and studying about human emotions over the last two-and-a-bit decades, as well as the privilege of being on the inside of other people's stories I can now see how both together have given me the narrative *and* the vocabulary of language that I have needed to ascribe language to my own experiences.

What I see from others without an insight into the inner worlds of autistic people, and what I read about autism and our emotional worlds, is so often steeped in the deficit-based, pathological notion that *all* autistic people don't feel emotion, or they lack empathy.

These assumptions and generalizations are made from what they see on the outside, not what is being experienced on the inside. And of course, not one autistic person is the same – we are all different. We are not a monolith, and every autistic person will experience their emotional world in their own unique way. As with any population, there are always differences in experiences.

'I did a postgrad in Emotional Education in 2019 which gave me the vocabulary to explore and express my emotions more effectively. I get very overwhelmed and sometimes furious if I observe or experience injustice.'

'Books, such as Daniel Goleman's *Emotional Intelligence* and Marc Brackett's *Permission to Feel* have been so helpful. I still experience a delay in understanding my emotions. I need days, sometimes weeks, to process so if I am asked "are you ok?" in the moment I will answer "yes" as a kneejerk reaction even if it is evident that I am struggling.'

Alexithymia

Perhaps some of those assumptions come from what we now understand is alexithymia – a term that you may or may not be familiar with. It was first introduced in the 1970s and loosely translates in Greek to mean 'no words for emotions'. Whilst alexithymia is not unique to autism, studies and research (Kinnaird *et al.*, 2020) show that it is more prevalent in the autistic community than the general population, and that alexithymia is common, rather than universal in autism, supporting a growing body of evidence that co-occurring autism and alexithymia represents a specific subgroup in the autistic population.

It can show up as having difficulties in identifying feelings, and in describing and expressing feelings to other people, amongst other things. For some autistic people, alexithymia may not feature or reflect their experience of their inner emotional world, but it may be something you want to explore further on your rediscovery journey. Some of our community members share their experiences which may or may not resonate with you:

'I struggle with showing emotions that are socially expected of me, there's always a processing lag until I find the right response and expression. It's like I'm going through a giant rolodex of emotions and facial expressions. I don't always get it right.'

'However, when I was in the corporate world, I found it good to have a rather blank emotionless persona – I had a great GAME face. Helped me navigate the politics – I never reacted in the moment as I was never sure how to react. So, I could go away and process things and be very deliberate in my reactions.'

'I struggle to disengage from my family's emotional states when I am around them. It is still a struggle to recognize my emotions in the moment, there is always a delay (getting better at this), processing takes time and journaling helps.'

'Reading/listening to other autistic people's experiences and emotions really shines a light on how I feel about/process my experiences. To my knowledge I don't know any autistic person apart from my own son. It is helpful to share and infodump in online chat groups.'

'I realize that showing simple things like pleasure at meeting a family member or friend have always been less in me than what I witness in others. And I think to a degree I put on a reaction, it does not emerge naturally or spontaneously.'

'So it does make me wonder about the authenticity of my relationships. The desire to be joyous and effusive is there, but I do not know how to let it out. The inner landscape of my body's tensions and rumblings is easier for me to read and realize "Ah, I am excited, sad, anxious".'

EXPLORING *YOUR* EMOTIONAL WORLD

Coming home means making sense of your own emotional world, looking within, connecting with your lifetime of lived experience, and giving yourself the permission to nurture yourself through self-knowing and self-understanding – only then do we start to feel like we are coming home.

A good place to start is to examine how you find identifying, understanding and describing your emotions. Consider how you find showing, expressing or feeling emotions that are socially expected of you.

Consider what you know helps you in processing and recognizing your emotions, and reflect on where or how you feel your emotions. Do you allow yourself the opportunity to consider 'why' you are feeling what you are feeling? How can you gently encourage more reflection?

Layered on all of this is how emotions were handled and approached in your family unit growing up. How do you think your family/childhood experience has shaped your beliefs about emotions? Were all emotions encouraged? Tears welcomed? How were your emotions received by your caregivers?

And a reminder that we are all different and all unique in terms of our life stories and how we experience the world. It's ok if you don't struggle to process your emotions, or if you are someone who isn't hyper-empathetic, we are not a monolith. Your rediscovery journey is about understanding *your* emotional world. What are your emotional strengths and struggles? That might mean asking others in your world who know you and who you trust to help fill in some of the gaps, or to offer a perspective you are unable to see about yourself.

The Frequency Circle in your Rediscovered Toolkit in Chapter 12 might be helpful for you here to explore what helps you dial into your own frequency.

CHAPTER 5

Our Cognitive World

This chapter focuses on how we experience our cognitive world, the way that our *monotropic minds dive to the deepest depths, our passionate interests and understanding your own unique cognitive world.* For far too long, the autistic experience has been framed as a deficit, especially when it comes to our cognitive style. I really dislike the term 'executive dysfunction' and the theory behind it, because it proposes that we have dysfunctional executive functioning, that we are broken in some way, not a fully functioning human being, when actually what we are talking about is a difference – a difference in the way our brains function from the neuronormative.

Defining autism as a difference doesn't take away or dismiss the struggles or challenges that an autistic person experiences, but there is a duality, because with struggles there are also strengths, and all too often we overlook strengths, or underplay support needs – people like to put us on a linear line of one or the other. But the two can and do co-exist, often referred to as our 'spiky cognitive profile'.

The first step in my own journey to rediscovery and compassionate acceptance of myself was working out the things I struggle with as well as identifying and understanding my cognitive strengths, and being brutally honest with myself about my struggles, and why I struggle. Much as with my sensory struggles, I find that if there is too much cognitive input to process my frequency quickly becomes scrambled.

My brain seeks safety in things and depends on (my) structure, (my) routine, predictability, familiarity and sameness in my daily life in order to reduce the cognitive load. I struggle with following instructions, planning ahead, packing to travel, menu planning – anything that involves forward planning is something that I really struggle with, and I can't tell you how many times I have got lost as an adult because I can't follow a map or follow step by step instructions, which is a large part due to co-occurring dyspraxia. It's as though I hit a brick wall in my head and the neuronal pathway that *should* be there hits a dead-end.

This was a particular struggle for me when I had to travel with work and would be given a set of instructions of where I had to be. There were many times when I would have to stop a police officer, and explain that I was lost in London and needed some help in finding my way to my hotel. Or the time that I went out running up one of the three Yorkshire Peaks and couldn't find my way home, lost until I stumbled across a group of potholers who thankfully got me back safely to my starting point – there are many more tales like these that I've felt mortifyingly embarrassed and ashamed about and this explains why I like familiarity and will revisit the same places over and over.

It took me seven attempts to pass my driving test, in one failed attempt I had gone the wrong way up a one-way street, I found having to listen to instructions whilst simultaneously *doing* too overwhelming, my mind struggles with following verbal sequences or steps, and I have a history of failing exams, because my memory recall always lets me down. The driving test story is just one in many situations I have struggled in my life, questioning why my brain can't show up for me the way it does for others.

My brain processes things very literally. I don't get sarcasm and most jokes are lost on me, which people have and do point out to me, repeatedly, especially when I don't give the response people deem to be the 'norm'.

My brain works on a 'now and next' basis – what I have to do now, and the need to know what's happening next, and whilst I don't lack imagination in many aspects of my world, I do find it hard to put myself into future scenarios – to think about what might happen next or what I might need in a future situation. Throughout my life that has meant getting myself into situations that have harmed me or set me up to fail, or I fail to plan and I'm unprepared in all sorts of situations.

If there are too many days to think about or too much information to consider, I go into cognitive overwhelm. That's why looking up, creating the big ideas, and visualizing the big-ticket stuff plays to my strengths. But it also means that I struggle with forward thinking beyond the now and next, something I found immensely stressful for the decade of my life that I was part of a blended family with not just my own life and diary to manage and navigate but having to plan around others too. It helped to have shared calendars and a group WhatsApp but I was drowning underneath the day to day planning. I've only recognized and acknowledged this now I'm no longer in it.

Packing to go away is something I find intensely difficult because I can't think about what I might want to wear a day in advance, never mind a week in advance, and I struggle to imagine what we might be doing, what the weather might look like, and so I end up taking everything, yet always forgetting something important. Sending birthday cards on time, filing my tax return, basic life admin and what we are going to eat for dinner are some of the life tasks I struggle with, yet I have this need to feel ordered and structured in all aspects of my life.

I was that person who in order to prepare for my autism assessment categorized and ordered my thoughts into pages and pages (and even more pages) of evidence. It was an exhausting process but my mind has to create structure and flow.

I'm definitely team words over team numbers. I hate maths with a passion, and statistics, and anything that has a string of multiple verbal instructions. I struggled massively with the quantitative research element in my psych Master's and failed my stats exam and couldn't bring myself to attempt to re-sit it. Yet I wrote a first class psych Master's thesis in less than a week, and achieved first class marks in my written work – work where I could be creative and was not being tested on my memory recall ability, and I discovered a passion for thematic analysis as a tool of finding patterns in narrative data.

My mind works in pictures, I'm a visual thinker and I have an eidetic memory – which comes from the Greek word that means 'seen'. I applied those strengths whilst writing this book because I can picture all the chapters visually in my head and I can lay them all out, and have a helicopter view of where the specific bits of content need to go and I can see the paragraphs in such detail in my mind.

I wrote the majority of this book in a four-week period sandwiched between my breast surgery recovery and radiotherapy treatment beginning, and I found that whilst I was driving or showering or sleeping that I would be coming up with content and slotting the data into the chapters laid out in my mind. I would have to pull over when I was driving to physically then slot the content into whichever chapter or paragraph it fit; these were structured and ordered in my google drive.

I'm also able to explain the most complex of things in a simple framework or picture, and I see patterns in people's stories. Being a visual thinker is a strength I am able to nurture in my work as a therapist and it's something I get to embrace in the therapy room, weaving my creative and very visual mind into my practice, and indeed as a storyteller. It's how I make sense of the world.

In my sessions that can look like drawing a picture, or describing something that is complex very visually and metaphorically, creating frameworks, paradigms, and using visual based narrative exercises to aid in self-discovery and self-understanding. All this helps the people who work with me to see things, the world, and themselves through a compassionate lens and different perspective.

It's a skill that supported me at the point of diagnosis with my breast cancer. Applying the 'mountain metaphor' aided me to make sense of, and give narrative to, my own journey of 'climbing the mountain'. When I lost control of my carefully constructed familiar and predictable world, the way I re-anchored myself was to draw a picture of the mountain I was about to climb and the basecamp tent I found myself in, waiting for the experts to find me the best route up the north face of the mountain, knowing that this team of experts would be with me every step of my climb, along with a team of sherpas who pledged to come on this climb with me.

Each chemo cycle meant another stage of the mountain climbed, and each hospitalization was a set-back due to poor weather, or acclimatization. On the days when I couldn't get out of bed, I was sheltering in place, with the knowledge that the snow would clear and the sun would shine once again, and when I was struggling mentally, physically and emotionally I imagined anchoring myself onto the north face of the mountain.

One of the things I observed during the two weeks that fell between my initial breast clinic appointment where I was told they were 99 per cent certain that I had breast cancer and me getting my diagnosis and treatment plan was how my mind needed to know what was coming next and so set about working out and extrapolating every possible route up the mountain to prepare myself for what was coming – from best to worst case scenario.

It was an exhausting two weeks, and meant that when I did meet with my oncologist for the first time and I was given the news and my route up the mountain that I felt prepared. What my oncologist saw from the outside was a Catherine who didn't show any outward emotion at the news, or seem fazed by what she was telling me – not a 'typical' reaction to what is life-changing news. But what she couldn't see, and what others don't see, are the internal workings of my mind and the depths I dived to in those previous two weeks to retune my frequency. Some might call it 'catastrophizing' – I call it 'regulating' and preparing myself for whatever route I was to be given.

I can feel the intensity of emotion in my body that will come once I've conquered this mountain that I've named Mount Cooke. A colourful print of this mountain hangs next to my bed so that each morning and each night I can visualize where I am at on my climb, and the colourful flag I will place to mark my climb – my beautiful autistic mind came to my rescue during what was, and still is, the most brutal climb of my life, and for that, I will forever be thankful.

My cognitive strengths

- Words as data
- Can spot patterns and themes in that data
- Creative writing
- Visual thinker with an eidetic memory
- Big thinker
- Idea generator
- My mind wants to go deep
- Compelling narrative and storytelling
- Connector of dots
- Can simplify complexity
- Likes to problem solve
- Space holder
- Community builder

My cognitive struggles

- Too many instructions, too many steps
- Too many words together
- Transitions from one task to another
- Doing more than one thing at once
- Verbal instructions
- Navigating and map reading
- Humour and jokes
- Too many demands

- Planning ahead
- Thinking on the spot
- Working out the time in a digital format
- Recalling the 'right' words
- Speech

Working out what makes my struggles worse

- Stress
- Burnout
- Menopause
- Lack of sleep
- Being in pain
- Feeling too hot
- Hunger
- Trauma

Working out what adaptations work for me (tunes back into my frequency)

- Voice notes (time to process)
- Now and next, not planning too far ahead
- Buffers of time between transitions
- Time blocking
- Picture clocks
- Assimilation time

- Lowering demands

- Space and solitude

- Spoken word shutdown/periods of not speaking and silence

- Scripting

- Routine and structure (mine, not someone else's)

- Predictability and familiarity (not intolerant of change, in fact I need change)

- Writing vs speaking

- Qualitative vs quantitative

- Assignments vs exams

- Time to process

- Small groups/1:1

- Safe environments

- Visual instructions and prompts

- Support with the things I struggle with

 EXPLORING *YOUR* COGNITIVE WORLD

Using the SASA Framework in Chapter 12, what have you noticed about your own cognitive strengths and struggles? It may be that you have never really given much thought to this, or that throughout your life the focus (from others and/or yourself) has always been on the things you struggle with which has overlooked your strengths.

Conversely, you may be so attuned to your strengths that you have never allowed yourself to actually consider the things that you struggle with cognitively. Spend some time now thinking about your cognitive strengths and struggles.

- What are your cognitive struggles and what are your cognitive strengths?

- It might be helpful here to ask trusted people around you. What do they see that you don't? Is there a blind spot you can't see?

- Have there been specific times or chapters in your life that have impacted on the things you struggle with?

- Can you name them? What can you identify that makes your cognitive struggles worse?

- What about things that have enabled you to play to your cognitive strengths? If you were to look back on your life would you say that you have known what your cognitive strengths are? Have you been able to design your life/career/work/ around your cognitive strengths?

- Now that you know your cognitive strengths and struggles, what can you identify that you need in terms of adaptations, and what adaptations have you already made in your life/ working world/family unit? Are there any other adaptations you now know you need to make to help you tune back into your frequency and come home to yourself?

- And now consider what you need from others around you. What accommodations can you seek out to help you tune into your frequency? These might be in the home, at work, within your day to day. Do you feel able to request these accommodations? If not, what do you recognize is a barrier or challenge for you? How can you overcome those barriers and challenges?

- Finally, I want you to imagine what it would look or feel like if you were able to strength nurture and support your struggles more in your life. What would that change for you?

- Go back to your SASA Framework. What do you need to seek out more from others to support you (accommodations) and what can you do to support yourself (adaptations)?

This exploration may hit you hard. You might realize that you have been underplaying or hiding your struggles, or that you have been 'pushing through' and masking the fallout. Or perhaps that you are finding it hard to focus on your strengths.

Bring your awareness here to one of compassion.

You are a human being, not a human 'doing', with a set of unique struggles and strengths. You are allowed to make adaptations and seek out accommodations on this rediscovered journey of yours.

Our ability to dive to the deepest of depths (AKA monotropism)

Monotropism is a term that was coined by (Murray *et al.*, 2005) to describe attention that focuses on a narrow range of interests, and for me it is a fundamental theory in our understanding of the autistic mind.

In a monotropic mind, fewer interests tend to be aroused at any time, and they attract more of our processing resources, making it harder to deal with things outside of our current attention tunnel. When I think of monotropism, I imagine a boat in the ocean. For those with a polytropic mind they are content with jumping into the sea, and having a leisurely swim, perhaps with others, before making their way back to the boat to soak up the sun and chat to others before heading back to shore.

In contrast, the montropic mind has a stronger pull and is preparing to deep dive, busy getting their wetsuit and diving gear on to be pulled into the deep depths of the ocean to marvel at the illuminating coral under the sea, in what is largely a solo expedition. There is no sense of time on the seabed, and no sense of urgency or end date to the dive, running out of oxygen the only real reason why the dive has to come to an end. It's a magical place of wonder and delight, a place where joy is found and our 'flow state' activated.

Through a neuro-affirming lens, what we see is monotropism often outwardly expressed as passion and unequivocal devotion to an area of study or research, an impressive and distinguished collection of items, or a formidable focus on a particular interest or sensory experience. I liken it to a kind of meditative state, writing this book doesn't feel like work, rather I am in deep flow, the kind where I lose my sense of time, and where my interoceptors are muted.

I will trade sleep for flow state, and be oblivious to the need to go to the toilet, drink, eat and take breaks unless someone puts those things in front of me, and I find it emphatically difficult to tear myself away from the harmony this flow state elicits in my brain. I imagine all my neurons are firing in synchronization – I'm transported to the image in my head of a synchronized swimming team, performing with the utmost grace in my mind when I'm in my deep dive expedition – why would I want that to end?

And whilst there's an urgency and 'hyperfocus' to my writing, it comes from the excitement of having spent so long immersed in the water, diving to the deepest depths of the ocean, going to places others haven't been and wanting to bring to the surface what I've found on these dives for others to share – this has now been my interest for several years and I'm ready to share with the world what I've learned and how I've made sense of it all in my own mind. A data cleanse so that I can reset and restore, making way for the next deep dive and book number two.

The first 10,000 words of this book were written over the space of a week, and once I'd formulated the idea for the book and secured the contract to publish it, I became driven and consumed with wanting to finish it, only to be given the news a few weeks after I committed to writing this book that I had breast cancer. Chemotherapy treatment started imminently and I wrongly assumed that I would continue to write throughout my treatment.

However, the reality of six months of chemotherapy was that I lost my ability to do anything other than put one foot in front of the other up the breast cancer mountain, and some days I couldn't even manage that – all I could do was shelter in place, and anchor myself into the north face of the mountain I was climbing. I wasn't in creative mode, or flow state, but survival mode, and my 'go to' interests where I experience joy and 'flow' were no longer accessible, which added an extra challenging layer to my already brutal treatment.

As my chemotherapy treatment came to an end and my surgery was completed, the mountain top was for the first time visible, and with the most challenging parts of my climb accomplished and behind me, my creativity and access to my flow state began to return, not to previous levels, but enough to allow me to deep dive again. The words (thankfully) began to flow.

I had a real sense of determination and commitment to use the window of less harsh conditions between treatments to bring this book to life. When you are faced with your own mortality, it highlights how the only time we really have is now, and I have so much I want to say and share with the world. I also recognize that these insights and knowledge I've collated on my deep dives have become too consuming for me to simply retain in my head and this book is about becoming less inward focused and more outward driven – I need to share this knowledge.

I think this was the solution to the inertia I felt trying to re-engage my flow after six months of no writing. I knew all I had to do was to imagine myself on that boat, in my diving suit, my feet in the water and to take the plunge to reconnect – and reconnect I did; before I knew it I was back on that ocean floor with an added layer of experience and a whole different perspective on life.

In stark contrast, the current diagnostic criterion for autism (American Psychiatric Association. DSM-5, 2017) instead pathologizes monotropism in the way it describes those outwardly expressed behaviours, and when autism is framed in such deficit-based language within the pathology paradigm, it's little wonder that there is so much stigma and shame linked to autism, and why mental health issues and suicide ideation are far more prevalent.

One of the challenges of monotropism is how it can, and does, lead to overwhelm and burnout, especially when we have to split our attention between diving and doing other things. When I wrote my psych thesis the only way I could complete it was to lock myself away in my office for a week. I needed as few distractions as possible and not to have to keep coming up to the surface, getting out of my diving gear, dried and back to shore on repeat. It's exhausting having to try and split my attention in this way without enough time to recharge (which for me looks like space, solitude and time to decompress) something that Adkin and Gray (2022) describe as 'monotropic split' which can lead to autistic burnout and mental health difficulties.

And whilst I was writing this book, there were distractions of work, of cancer treatment, of being mum, of healing and recovering from my treatment. I have found that time blocking helps me mitigate and minimize the impact of monotropic split now that I have this self-knowledge. Dedicating a chunk of time to my interest (my book) – time when I won't be interrupted or pulled away – is an adaptation I can make for myself, and an accommodation I can seek out from others to accommodate my way of working.

Monotropism, and the monotropic split, explains autistic people's challenges with inertia and switching between tasks when we are immersed in our deep dives and graciously skimming the ocean floor – it leaves little attention for what is happening on the surface. Monotropism can and does also bring with it a deep sense of loneliness, of otherness, of sitting on the periphery and never really feeling like you belong on the surface. I find it hard to watch anything, to give my attention to something unless I'm hooked, and when I'm hooked it becomes all consuming, like binge watching the entire series of *Game of Thrones* in the space of a month. I can see how that might be perceived as being too 'intense' or 'obsessive' and why addiction is so prevalent amongst the autistic community.

Our monotropic minds are also a strength, a truly powerful force for creativity, and what we find as we deep dive into the ocean depths is life we wouldn't see on the water's surface, and that leads me to reconsider the concept of 'rest' in this context. My interests are where I'm most happy, yet on the outside that looks like 'doing'. I know that when I put my deep dive suit on and the oxygen mask goes on that I get to explore places I can't see or access on the surface; it's just a different form of rest.

Not being able to engage in it during my cancer treatment put me into a state of under-stimulation and under-arousal, I felt restless, distressed and anxious and I found myself having to develop new interests to enable me to continue to dive, an exhausting interest which became knowing and learning everything I could about my type of breast cancer and my treatment.

I have this relentless internal energy that never stops, and whilst from the outside looking in that might look like 'drive' and has been described as that many times, it's actually an all-consuming inner energy that pre-discovered me was oblivious to. My interoceptive needs weren't heard to the point of burnout and chronic ill health, because I get drawn into such singular focus that I neglect my basic needs.

I remember telling a friend about my late discovery and she responded by saying she could see that by how I never stand still, I'm always doing the next project and how exhausting that must be. That depth and pull of my monotropic mind is both a strength and a challenge. However, the joy I am able to tap into when I reach those depths, and the things that my mind has created and brought to life from those dives, that's a very special skill and feeling that I get to experience which I now know isn't universally experienced.

There's a lesson here, a piece of nature wisdom, because oceans don't ever apologize for their depth. People marvel at the ocean; they sit for hours. Imagine the ocean marvelling back at you in the same way.

What would that change for you?

But also we benefit from having the knowledge now that if we push our autistic brains to operate and perform in a polytropic way, what inevitably happens is outcome overwhelm. When our brains consume more than they are able to process at any one time, the outcome is that it scrambles our frequency.

Is there any wonder then that our bodies scream enough and we bungee jump into autistic burnout, crash our way into shutdown or become paralyzed and detached from ourselves by the lack of monotropic stimulation? And isn't this also why at certain transition points or touch points in our lives when we find ourselves in situations where we are unable to deep dive we struggle more?

Monotropism as a theory is not just helpful for us as late

discovered autistic women to create the environment we need in which to thrive, it's also a helpful theory for our loved ones and anyone we share an environment with. Being an ally looks like being able to recognize how to nurture that and how to support that is a game changer. Taking an interest, supporting, understanding, enabling and space giving matters.

Passionate interests

When it comes to our interests, I prefer to think of them as 'passions' rather than pathologizing them as 'special' or 'obsessions' – language matters. Our interests aren't 'weird' or 'too much', they are where we find our joy. I read non-fiction, prefer real life stories to imaginary ones, have never got comedy, and struggle to watch anything that isn't deeply engaging and emotional, or science fiction, second world war or apocalyptic themed.

I've had a 25-year love affair with all things psychology, people and human behaviour. Over the last decade I've refined that to having a deep interest in women's' mental health and wellbeing, and, more recently, late discovered autism. I've wrapped my career around my interests which means I find joy, meaning and purpose in my work.

My favourite place in the world is Copenhagen, and I am drawn to the ice kingdoms of the north. Once I've finished my book and my cancer treatment, I'd like to spend more time exploring and learning about Scandi culture and why it's so appealing to my neurodivergent mind, and I have an impressive collection of colourful hats and coats that I like to categorize and organize by colour, red lipstick, statement earrings and books.

In the early part of my childhood we lived around the corner from an athletics stadium, and both my parents were avid runners and ran competitively. From being young I ran for our local running club, and after a break as a teenager, picked back up my passion for running during my 20s, and it became something I had to do every day, often running 40+ miles a week and always pushing myself to run further and enter races.

Running solo, with my music on, in nature was pure heaven for me and where I found my flow, and whilst it's no longer an interest or something I can do, I look back with a full heart and gratitude that I was able to experience that depth of joy.

My mum's passion was swimming, she dedicated her childhood and teens to the sport, and was training for the national team until breaking her arm playing leapfrog put an end to her professional swimming ambition, and meant she *taught* swimming rather than competed. It was my mum who got me hooked into swimming from being a baby, and even now it's one of the many joys I experience when I'm gliding through the water.

I'm thankful that swimming was never pushed or commodified into having to train or do lessons, rather it became something I associated with tuning into my frequency. In my meditation practice I am often transported in my mind to the swimming pool that I spent my early childhood swimming in and it's a passion I've introduced to my girls, and an activity we can share together. There is something about the rhythmic nature of lane swimming, and tuning down the senses with goggles and ear plugs that centres me – it's a self-regulating, sensory soothing, flow activating activity I can access and I'm so grateful to my mum for that gift.

We are lifelong learners and I find wonder and delight in knowing that there is still so much to explore, and when I discover other people who too need that depth, and come alive when they go to those depths, and want to dive with me, or talk about their dives and what they find and how much joy it brings them – well, that's pure autistic magic, and I'm here for the magic.

If there's one single important aspect of our autistic neurology that needs nurture and understanding it's to allow our passionate interests to guide the way. Channelling our monotropic minds and diving deep into our passionate interests is the equivalent of applying a soothing balm to our nervous system.

Being able to deep dive is where we find our most joy, and here some of The Late Discovered Club Community share their passions and specific interests.

'My special interest is breastfeeding. I read something really interesting recently about how many neurodivergent breastfeeding mothers end up with it becoming a special interest due to facing challenges with it and then become obsessed with fixing it – I couldn't just breastfeed, I had to become an expert and get a qualification!'

'I've always loved animals, and now we have 16 pets – dogs, cats, tortoises, ferrets and giant snails. Giant snails (actually any snails) have always been a passion of mine. I used to sneak garden snails up to my room and keep them in random containers. My parents kept finding them under the bed. I still get excited when I see snails out and about. At one point I had about 40 giant snails of different species, few people got that, definitely a "special" interest.'

'My interests are in art, textiles, nature, mushrooms and SEND. Being in the natural world is very important to me – but I need to look at it through a lens of creativity, i.e. natural dyes, earth pigments, lake pigments, wild inks, foraging, fibres and cordage.'

'My interests are in all that has and is evolving from body-mind centring practices. The feeling of embodiment from somatic yoga and embodied flow yoga which leads into an ability to try other movement modalities and dance workshops.'

'The joyous sense of being immersed in such music as Olafur Arnalds and seeing where the movement takes me. I am hooked. And swimming – my son taught me front crawl when I was 65. I love the feel of the movement and my flow through the water.'

'My special interests have covered a wide array of themes, ranging from rocks when I was little, to musical theatre, feminist theories and gender studies, different chapters of world history, video games such as animal crossing, books by specific authors such as Isabel Allende, among many other topics. Unfortunately, I have dropped many special interests along the way because of social pressure and silly attempts to "fit in" or stop being "so weird or intense".'

'Puzzles – very cliche I know, but they've been something I've done religiously since a small child. They enable me to switch off from the world, I can get so absorbed and sit for hours without realizing the time. I also love documentaries on planes and airports, trains, any kind of travel. Japan – never been but obsessed. Exercise. If I don't do something most days I get twitchy.'

'Music, words and language, nature, photography, the sea, culture (art, poetry, books). My kids became a special interest when I became a mother, I don't know how I would have coped with the challenges of motherhood otherwise. Autism has become a special interest, right now I am deep diving synaptic pruning.'

 ### EXPLORING *YOUR* DEEP DIVES AND PASSIONATE INTERESTS

To help you explore your deep dives and passionate interests I want to bring your awareness to the here and now. What is it that brings you joy? What is/are your current passionate interests? Are you in a season of your life currently where you are able to deep dive?

- Has there ever been a time in your life when you've been

unable to access your passionate interests or perhaps where you've not been able to deep dive as much as you need to? What do you recognize about those times?

- If you are struggling right now to name your passionate interests I want you to now shift your awareness to the younger version of you. Looking back at your childhood, what were your passionate interests? Were your interests supported by your caregivers/in your education environment?

- And now bring your awareness back to the last time you were in monotropic flow, when you are skimming the surface of the ocean floor, how does that make you feel? What do you notice that can happen when you are in full monotropic flow?

- What do you need others in your life to know? To be aware of or to help you with?

- What do you need to do more/less of in order to access that magical joy going forwards?

- What does 'rest' look like for you?

CHAPTER 6

The Places We Go to When the World Feels Too Much

*Content warning: In this chapter I talk about suicide.

How we respond, and the places we go to when the world feels too much are, without doubt, some of our most painful and shameful parts of being autistic. The meltdowns, shutdowns and what I like to term 'overspills' are enshrined in guilt, embarrassment and humiliation along with a heavy serving and burden of shame, which links to feelings of unworthiness, and the deprivation of belonging and acceptance – our mental health bearing the nuclear level fall out.

Hearing out loud the many stories and experiences through the space of the The Late Discovered Club Circles, and within our wider community, what I've learned is that as women we've been socially conditioned from a such young age to find other (more socially acceptable) ways of responding when the world feels too much, and that these don't always 'look' like the 'fight' response that we read and hear about, or generally associate with an autistic meltdown, but rather the flight, freeze, fawn and flop response, and often hidden from view.

The sheer level of resilience that it has taken to live our lives in this way has gone unremarkably unnoticed, by others and indeed ourselves. All the times we've reached our sensory, emotional, cognitive, social and relational tipping points, when our neurology can't take any more input become the only moments that go noticed, moments that are seen clearly and judged heavily. The message we have heard loud and clear is one of needing to be 'more resilient' because we are 'too sensitive' when in fact we have been wearing the badge of resilience for as long as we can remember.

Unveiling shame

As late discovered women and people, our voices and experiences have been censored from the narrative that is out there. Talking about something that is so powerfully shame-inducing is a taboo for many, but by shining a light in this chapter on some of our most shameful experiences, the hope is that it empowers you to do the same, because shame dies in the light.

I hope that this chapter helps you feel seen, heard and understood, and by sharing the dark parts of our stories that have been veiled in shame, it empowers you to show yourself the self-compassion and gentle understanding you need and deserve, and to begin unveiling the shame that has consumed you, and silenced you up until now.

One of the things that has kept me going up the breast cancer mountain is the knowledge that even in our darkest of moments and our hardest of days, there is always the hope (and the delight) that the sun will rise on a brand new day. And with that new day, comes another layer of self-knowing.

We are all a work in progress, and you are no exception.

As you navigate this new world, take the time to look up and around, and stand proud.

Shame has no place in your rediscovered world, and the more self-compassion, self-understanding and self-kindness you can extend to yourself, the less available oxygen shame has to breathe in to keep itself alive.

From the inside out

A poem I wrote to describe the inner experience of the places we go to when our world feels too much.

Too much noise, too many different noises, too many voices.
Not enough space, silence or solitude.

Too many people, too much peopling, too much speaking.
Not enough time to prepare, script, recover and reset.

Too much clutter, too many eyes, too much stuff.
Not enough visual peace or calm.

Too many demands and too many distractions.
Not enough alone time, deep diving time, decompression time,
or restorative sleep.

Too much to process.
Not enough time or space to process it.

Too many pressures and too many expectations.
Not enough energy or capacity.

Too much chaos and uncertainty.
Not enough predictability, structure or routine.

Too much heat.
Not having the time to regulate my temperature.

Too much structure to the point of feeling repressive and
trapped.
Not enough flexibility or room to breathe.

Too much conformity, imposed structure or changes without
communicating.
Not enough agency, choice or autonomy.

Too much communication, too many words, too much talking.
Not enough alternative modes of communicating.

Too many differing needs.
Not being able to prioritize my own needs.

Too much ambiguity.
Not enough planning or preparation.

Too much judgement, too many assumptions and
misunderstanding.
Not enough kindness.

Too much feeling like an outsider, or that I've done something
wrong.
Not enough empathy and understanding.

The emotion and distress internalizing.
Our inner voice growing louder.
A fire roaring within.
The overwhelm builds.
Pushing it down, holding back the tide, pressing the override
button on our nervous system until the system is breached.
What comes are tears, overspills, meltdowns, shutdowns and
eventually burnout and physical pain as we respond to a world
that feels too much.

This last sentence that I've highlighted is the bit that people often see. Not all of it, perhaps just a small part of it. Meltdowns are often the extent to which autism is viewed, defined and understood by people from the outside looking in. The behaviours of 'concern' and 'challenging' behaviours that people see and wrongly assume *is* autism. It's the behaviour we are judged on, and the behaviour we judge ourselves on.

'They make me feel extremely embarrassed to be honest. I think they completely change other people's perception about me as a person in a very stigmatizing way.'

From the outside in

According to the National Autistic Society (NAS, 2024), an autistic meltdown is defined as 'an intense response to an overwhelming sensory or emotional stimuli'. The Autism Research Institute (ARI, 2024) offers a further definition which describes meltdowns as 'involuntary responses to a nervous system overload. They are the physical manifestation of neurobiological chaos and are not behavioural responses and generally aren't used to attain a specific outcome'.

'Meltdowns tend to happen when I am emotionally overstimulated and shutdowns when I am overstimulated sensorially. The worst meltdown I have had since being diagnosed, and possibly ever, happened because I was about to have a week off work during which I was going to be turning 30 and which I thought/hoped I would be getting engaged.'

'I couldn't handle the mixture of excitement and uncertainty and this led to a meltdown. During this meltdown I smashed a plate and then punched myself in the head repeatedly. My partner had to restrain me to stop me, and he said I was screaming as if in pain as well as crying and repeatedly apologizing.'

'Meltdown feels like a civil war between my body and my mind. I fight to put out the fire but if I am dysregulated and then something additional happens to trigger me (some sort of sensory overwhelm). I can end up shouting, slamming doors, throwing things, punching things (always on my own). Shutdown feels like plunging into pitch-black abyss. Being dragged by my feet deep underwater, hopeless, suffocating and inescapable.'

'As a child I used to hit my head against the wall and bite my arms to externalize the pain when I was triggered. This childhood memory lay buried for years, I only remembered this once I was diagnosed. Even now, self-harm seems like a very reasonable option when battling the overwhelm of a meltdown, but I don't act on it.'

Research undertaken by a team at Stanford University (Supekar *et al.*, 2013) over a decade ago suggested that autistic people have neurons that are more hyper-connected than people who aren't autistic. The researchers used neuroimaging to show there are 'more instances of greater functional connectivity in the brains of children who are autistic compared with typically developing children'. This then perhaps explains why meltdowns and/or shutdowns feature prominently in our late discovered stories – our sensory systems are different, our neurotypes are different, and when the world feels too much meltdown and/or shutdown follows.

Shutdowns could be considered the mirror opposite to a meltdown, with our emotions focused inwards. Just like an iPhone goes into battery saving mode before it completely loses its power, and you lose the brightness and functionality, in autistic shutdowns our body goes into a battery saving mode too, prioritizing the basic functions, and shutting down other parts.

In autistic shutdown our ability to process input and information is reduced. That might look like spoken word and/or cognitive shutdown, curling up in a ball on the ground, leaving the space you are in, covering your face, shutting yourself away in a quiet space, being unable to make eye contact and not being able to communicate what is happening or why.

For me personally, my overspills and shutdowns largely happen internally and out of sight with my 'flight' response helpfully kicking in to get me out of the situation I'm in and to safety, an override button I've discovered I press until safety is reached, at which point the nervous system is breached and the tsunami of tears (the overspill) is unleashed and the shutting down happens. My internal verbal condemnation and tongue-lashing not directed to anyone but myself, and all within the confines of my own head.

'Shutdowns for me are a powering down, and a retreat from the world. It's an inability for me to speak, to join in, exhaustion and a crushing need to retreat to my own space. Meltdowns are anger, frustration, and spilling out. I'm shouty and a really bad version of myself. I sometimes feel the need to lash out, but more likely to run. To just get away and quickly. And then come the tears. Shutdown is the most frequent place I go to when the world feels too much.'

'As a parent of three young kids I'm quite often in environments or situations where I feel like everything has been physically drained out of me, and I need to go away and recharge. Days when I have to extreme multitask – mother, work, clients and lots of calls – then I'm generally speechless and spaced out.'

'I have lived by myself for many years and I now see that it has been relatively easy for me to remove myself from social engagement, activities/events or to increasingly say no when asked to go somewhere. I see now that this was shutdown – a non-engagement, protective way of removing myself and living alone in the safe space of my home.

Because of the way I do not understand emotions in myself or others I have gone into freeze rather than meltdown which I remember happening in my 20s. And freeze readily becomes shutdown.'

'In a shutdown, my body becomes so tense that I feel frozen, rooted to the spot. I feel muted, on pause – as though I can't speak or think. I can't take action. Meltdowns come out verbally for me. I lose control of what I'm saying and erupt with a tirade of hyperbolic, usually aggressive, words that I don't mean. I don't know what I'm saying or where the words come from, but it feels like a much-needed release; an emotional clear-out. I feel intense shame afterwards. Sometimes I'll throw things too – I've broken a few cups during meltdowns.'

Red flag events

My overspills and shutdowns are a nervous system red flag event. I imagine that inside my brain I have a carefully weaved internal alarm system present in each and every neuron. When the alarm sounds it's because I'm dangerously close to breaching a system overload. It signals to me that there is too much lighting up of my neurons in my head, be that emotional, cognitive or sensory, it's a code that I'm dysregulated and that the environment I'm in is no longer safe – the places, spaces and faces are at risk of overwhelming me.

I recognize that in my world, my shutdowns generally go unnoticed from the outside looking in and that, left unchecked, my shutdowns become the ringleaders to eventual burnout and ill health. Shutdowns are my battery saving mode – my world has to be dialled down, and I have an increasing need for alone time with my speech and social, emotional and cognitive functionality and ability significantly reduced.

I've also discovered that the key to downsizing them is through self-knowing and self-attunement of our own individual frequency, along with seeking out accommodations from others for all those things that sit outside of our control. Accommodation requests are not 'nice to do's' or 'should do's' for others to consider doing for the autistic people in their lives, rather they are 'must do's'. They are the aids and supports we need to help us tune into our frequency and find that equilibrium in all those environments we have little to zero control in.

The danger zone

We know that meltdowns and shutdowns have the ability to breach our sensitive nervous system and potentially take us into the danger zone, and when our nervous systems are engulfed by emotion and dysregulation, we might find ourselves in that moment *ideating* that *the only way* out of this danger zone is through closing the book on our story.

One of the hacks I have found that helps me in moments of overspill and shutdowns is to write it out. Write out everything I'm feeling in that moment, honestly and truthfully, and then immediately dispose of it once I'm on the other side. Not only does the mere process of writing out what's in my head act as a clearing tool (I imagine it's like a snowplough blasting through a snow laden road), it also simultaneously distracts me.

But equally having a safe person who can hold space and listen to the tears, fears and my internal monologue of condemnation without judgement and without interruption works just as well. Post overspill or shutdown, one of the kindest things I can do for myself is to allow myself to sleep – there's something so humanly healing about giving our minds and our nervous systems the opportunity to recover and reset through sleep, bathing our minds in our very own natural mood stabilizer that is serotonin. Things always seem more hopeful and less intense after a nap or a long sleep.

What also helps me is the knowledge I have about *what* it is I'm experiencing and *why*, along with all the helpful insights I have gained through self-knowledge and the learning from others that I never had access to before. As well as minimizing the triggers wherever possible to prevent future overspills and shutdowns.

One of the most profound books I have read that has added to this knowledge was *When It Is Darkest* (O'Connor, 2021). The book brings together decades of his work on suicide prevention at the University of Glasgow and it sheds light on why suicide happens, what you can do to prevent it, and how important it is to have a safety plan for if or when you find yourself in that dark place. Professor O'Connor says on the back cover of his book that 'one person dies by suicide every 40 seconds. But sadly, for the most part, we are reluctant to talk about it. It's one of the last remaining taboos'.

And whilst Professor O'Connor's work tells us that whilst one person dies by suicide every 40 seconds, one at-risk group that is still largely overlooked when it comes to this crisis is autistic people. A number of research studies have been compiled and outlined in a plan 'Meeting the needs of autistic adults in mental health services' (NHS England, 2023) including the research of Dr Sarah Cassidy at the University of Nottingham, which tells us that autistic people are:

> six times more likely to attempt death by suicide – and up to seven times more likely to die by suicide – compared to those who are not autistic. This risk of death by suicide is even greater among autistic people *without* intellectual disabilities, and when we apply an intersectional lens the risks become even higher. The greatest risk is actually among late discovered autistic women, who are 13 *times* more likely to die by suicide than women who are not autistic.

Researchers are not entirely clear why autistic people are at increased risk of having suicidal thoughts and behaviours, though it's likely a number of factors are at play, but maybe that lack of insight is because our experiences and insights as late discovered autistic women have never been heard. Inside the sanctuary of The Late Discovered Club Post Discovery Circles these experiences *are* heard and shared.

There is so much more support that could and should be offered to late discovered autistic women in terms of suicide prevention, including safety plans for when it is darkest. These should be a part of everyone's toolkit, spaces to speak out loud and hear others' experiences, as well as guidance to help ourselves understand our risks and triggers, and how we can reduce and mitigate them. And any professional who is working with/or person who is living with an autistic person needs to be aware and understanding of the risks and how to support when the world becomes too much, without judgement, with compassion, and in a trauma informed way.

We need and we deserve understanding and allyship.

What is clear, is that we need to power progress for late discovered autistic women and the high suicide risk that is associated with late discovery. Not just for those who have been able to access a formal diagnosis but for all those women who self-identify.

In Chapter 12 I share my Path of Self-Knowing exercise to help you better understand and make sense of your meltdowns and shutdowns, and the Frequency Circle may also come in useful here to help you understand the code to your own individual frequency, and importantly how you can become more attuned to it, and rediscover your own equilibrium, finding your centre of the circle in a world that we feel too much.

There is also my SASA framework to help you be in equal parts strengths focused and needs led, and in turn, better able to make the adaptations, and seek out the accommodations and support you need to help you thrive.

Trigger points

Autistic overspills, meltdowns and shutdowns can be triggered by many things. This is by no means a complete list, but it does reflect some of the most common triggers reported amongst our community:

- Sensory overload

- Emotional overload

- Things not happening as predicted/expected

- Cumulative trauma triggers

- The feeling that we've done something wrong or let someone down

- Not feeling safe

- Bullying, abuse, othering and people generally being unkind

- When things feel unjust

- Too much social interaction, too much to process and too many demands

- Feeling out of control in situations

'Sensory overload, being triggered back to traumatic times, being around people who are not emotionally safe for me, where I feel that I can't be/don't feel safe to be myself.'

'When I feel out of control and don't know what's going on, not being able to understand how a situation will make me feel or suddenly being in something I knew I wouldn't like but couldn't get out of. And then sometimes I'm in a bad mood and people (my family) keep going at me until I explode. They need to learn the signs. I regularly say when I know I'm on the edge "stop talking to me" but people don't and it gets worse.'

'Mainly social interaction but also being touched, too much noise and actually things not going to plan. Having a child has definitely tested me there.'

'Combinations of sensory overload and emotional spiralling. Feeling unfairly criticized, inadequate, misunderstood, misjudged, patronized by someone's actions or comments. If I feel unappreciated or invisible, ignored or sidelined that makes me intensely insecure which can lead to shutdown.'

And these are some of the factors that our community report that intensifies them:

- Prolonged or acute periods of stress

- Periods of change and big life transitions

- Grief and loss

- Pain

- Lack of sleep

- Hormones (puberty, pregnancy, post-natal, perimenopause, menopause)

- Burnout

- Being in the late discovery process

'They intensified during my late discovery. The development of knowledge and understanding of myself, my unmasking. Feelings flew and intensified through this time. I think masking has contained, hidden and dampened down overwhelm and shutdown. Since my mask has lifted I do feel emotions and often with great intensity. Paradoxical I guess!?'

'At university, while I was struggling with living in shared accommodation, with very little control over my home environment. Also, during the beginning of perimenopause, I've been more prone to meltdowns.'

'Times of huge transition and reckoning which have left me confused, vulnerable and lonely – leaving home, adapting to the workplace after university, becoming a mother (I think I probably had postpartum depression after both births), losing my dad, perimenopause/menopause years, seeing my son struggle with anxiety and depression, rejection from my husband, spite, criticism and impatience from my mother.'

'I feel like I experienced lots of meltdowns during pregnancy (hormones maybe played a part) but also I think because I remember feeling so weird and not comfortable having something growing inside me. I was very on edge and anxious.'

'And since having children. Three boys, all autistic, ADHD and various other things is a recipe for disaster as they trigger me daily, I probably trigger them too. And I very rarely get space and time to decompress and regulate. If I try to go upstairs and be by myself in the evening, I get told I'm unsociable. I can't win.'

Sending out an SOS

Meltdowns, overspills and shutdowns don't happen because we are broken.

They don't happen because we are less than.

They don't happen because we are 'lacking in self-control', or because we are 'drama queens' or 'too demanding'.

And they don't happen because we aren't fully functioning human beings.

They happen because our neurotypes are different to the neuronormative – we feel the world too much and we become overloaded.

If you are reading this book as someone who wants to know how best to support someone you know, love or care for when the world feels too much for them, the starting point is to ask them, listen and respond with love, kindness and compassion. Be guided by the autistic person in front of you, not what you 'think' you know. Accommodate and honour their needs, especially when they are signalling to you that they are in distress and need space, solitude and silence to regulate themselves.

Some of the members of our late discovered community share here what helps them when the world feels too much:

'Taking some time out on my own to breathe, and focus on how I'm feeling – ideally walking or driving to help regulate me.'

'Time, change of location, being alone, journaling, understanding why I feel triggered. Now I am learning to try and share my experience if I feel rejected or unappreciated and hopefully get some understanding and reassurance from my partner.'

'I talk to myself a lot. Sometimes out loud. I no longer allow my inner voice to subject me to constant criticism. Much as I know this is important, I still find recognizing and expressing my needs/vulnerabilities really hard given that I grew up treading lightly and being as undemanding as possible.'

'If it's an overwhelm/shutdown then going up to my office and reading or doing a puzzle (anything where I have to focus) either clears my head, or sometimes allows me to doze off and I always wake up feeling better.'

'If I'm out and about then putting on some noise cancelling headphones and listening to my special playlist brings everything back down and recharges. I often go out for a stomp and a listen and find that really helps with regulation. I quite often talk to myself and work through everyone's perspective out loud to figure things out while I walk.'

'The more I am, and can be my unmasked self it becomes easier, less of a challenge. Being with people who see and accept me for who I am, who get me. Being rested, fed, in a balanced mental and physical state. My nervous system being regulated and me recognizing that I am in a settled ok state.'

'If I do not feel ok, adjust what I do – taking a step back, lean with my back to a wall, let my breathing settle and my body feel grounded. Scan the environment to reassure myself that I am safe. I have learnt to listen and have heard how my body is attuned to the changing of the seasons. This has led to a rooted sense of my being in this world, on this planet.'

'For meltdowns, having my partner there to make sure I am safe helps (when possible). Having a bath helps for both meltdowns and shutdowns, as does lying on my bed with the fan on me listening to a favourite old audiobook or scrolling mindlessly on my phone.'

Lifesaving label

People often question why an autism diagnosis or self-identifying is needed if you are late discovered, or question why you need to give yourself a 'label' when you've got this far in life. Or we hear from well-meaning professionals that 'we are more than our labels' and not to create an entire identity around the label. For me, 'the label', without doubt, saved my life and changed my life.

That 'label' has given me a frame of reference and a depth of understanding I never had access to.

That 'label' has enabled me to show myself the empathy, self-compassion and kindness that I have needed for four whole decades.

That 'label' has facilitated the expansion of my self-knowing.

That 'label' has connected me to another world where our neuro-minority is a common humanity and with it, I've found acceptance, belonging and community.

That 'label' has enabled me to come home to myself.

It's not a 'label' that I self-apply to myself, rather it's an intrinsic part of who I am. It's not something I can choose to be or not to be.

I am autistic.

I identify as autistic.

I've always been autistic.

I will always be autistic.

 EXPLORING THE PLACES *YOU* GO TO

There is a distinct scarcity of understanding when it comes to the internalized world of autistic meltdowns, overspills and shutdowns, not just within our own family units, social circles and work environments, but right across those groups of professionals who work with autistic people, and more generally within our wider society.

And for those of us who have flown firmly under the autism radar (despite the lived experience) we too never had the narrative or the frame to help make sense of our own experiences prior to our late discovery.

Meltdowns and shutdowns are a uniquely personal and heavily shameful experience, and it was imperative to me to give voice to others from our Late Discovered Community to share their experiences in this chapter of what a meltdown and shutdown looks and feels like to them; to explore what their triggers are; to learn what intensifies them, and crucially, what helps.

These are experiences that, up until now, have been shamed into silence – they've never been heard before and are missing from the dataset. My hope is that the courage and compassion shown by the late discovered women who have opened up their books to share their inside story with you become the lights of hope on your own dark runway and that it makes exploring the places that you go to a less painful and shameful experience.

In the safety of your own journal perhaps you now feel ready to begin exploring what a meltdown and/or shutdown feels like for you? We've heard some very descriptive experiences in this chapter, how would you describe yours?

- What do you think triggers your meltdowns and/or shutdowns? If you allow yourself to reflect, are there any commonalities?

- Have there been any points in your life where they have intensified and/or become more frequent?

- What helps you? This might be a painful question to ask yourself because perhaps growing up your caregivers were unable to accommodate the things that actually help you. Perhaps you were denied access to the help you needed. This is where extra compassion towards yourself is needed. Ask yourself what it is you need?

As you embark on your own self-exploration over in Chapter 12 there is an additional, more in depth 'path of self-knowing' exercise to guide you in forensically examining and understanding your meltdown and shutdown experiences.

CHAPTER 7

When the Body Screams Enough

'Burnout feels like a complete lack of energy combined with a sense of a complete lack of control over any aspect of my life. My executive functioning gets worse, my sensory sensitivity and emotional dysregulation get worse and I have more meltdowns and/or shutdowns. It feels like everything is too hard and I've found myself back at square one.'

Living in a world that really isn't designed or accommodating of our neurotype is exhausting and can, and does, lead to autistic burnout, and not in the singular sense either. For many of us burnout has been an unwanted guest in our lives for as far back as we can remember – a perpetual cycle of overload, exhaustion, and the subsequent withdrawal from our lives as we know it, a distinct mismatch of demands vs resources, and all too often experienced on a physical level, with our bodies screaming enough.

If I were to try and visually describe what being in the trenches of autistic burnout looks and feels like, I'd tell you that it's like opening the door to your house to see that everything has been stripped out, with only the shell remaining.

All the things that brought joy are no longer there. In terms of recovery, bit by bit, every facet of your home has to be replaced, and replenished, and it takes time. We can't go back to how it was – what went before can't come again – and sometimes the very foundations of our house have borne the brunt and need reinforcing and rebuilding – there's a sense of having to put yourself back together, but each time also having to take things away, decluttering by removing our stressors, stripping out the social elements, and a stepping back.

We have to become fierce protectors and guardians of our energy – our worlds often becoming smaller as a consequence, and change is the only constant when it comes to burnout recovery. When our bodies scream enough, it's no longer battery saving mode we are entering, it's a signal that the way we are living our life *has* to change.

There is very little to no research out there about autistic burnout in late discovered women and even less research about the psycho immunological connection between autistic burnout and chronic pain, illness, cancer and all the other ways that burnout wreaks havoc on our bodies – despite it being one of the universally collective experiences I have heard our community bond over – which means that there is little to no professional knowledge and technical 'know how' when it comes to assessment, treatment, prevention and recovery.

Unsurprisingly then, it's clear to see why it's wholly misunderstood by health professionals who will mistake and mislabel autistic burnout for depression (amongst other things), especially when so many women are unable to access an autism diagnosis and why the dots aren't being connected. However, there has been some encouraging new research undertaken (Arnold *et al.*, 2023) at the University of New South Wales in Sydney, Australia, which focused on the development of an assessment tool to enable the identification and diagnosis of autistic burnout.

Whilst their research didn't focus specifically on late discovered autistic women, they did survey 141 autistic adults with experience of burnout in order to identify the factors that are associated with severity, develop an autistic burnout assessment and test the pre-publication of the AASPIRE Autistic Burnout Measure tool.

The findings from their research highlighted 'a core phenomenon, comprising exhaustion, withdrawal and cognitive overload, associated with stressors potentially unique to autistic people'. Furthermore, how long and how often people get autistic burnout was not clear. Participants told the researchers that they have:

> both short and long episodes and that autistic burnout leads to exhaustion, and that they needed to withdraw from being with other people and stay away from autism unfriendly places. Many had been misdiagnosed as having depression, anxiety, bipolar disorder, borderline personality disorder or other conditions.

What was clear to the researchers who undertook this study was that 'we need increased awareness of autistic burnout. Autistic people need more help. More research is needed, and we need to have bigger studies to understand autistic burnout.' Yet within our Late Discovered Community we know what autistic burnout is, and what it feels like because we've been living it and experiencing it for decades.

'It's the removal of myself from the world of people. In the past I have used illness such as a cold or virus as an excuse to others to say no and stay at home. Extending this to several weeks of avoidance until I recovered enough to be around people again.'

'Maybe in my late discovery there is a possibility of this changing. To tell others what is really going on with me. And the possibility that I will not get to the point of such profound burnout. I know what takes me there now.'

'For me it's physical illness – UTIs , pyelonephritis, acalculous cholecystitis (until my gallbladder was removed), headaches, fatigue, dyshidrotic eczema and anxiety. It feels awful – at its worst I've ended up in hospital, but then at least I feel I have permission to rest, because if I'm in hospital rest is allowed.'

'Like I'm walking through sticky mud – hard to move forward, but if I stop, I'll sink. Exhausted down to my bones, empty and hollow, but also feeling like lead. On autopilot – as tired as I am I can keep getting up and going.'

'Physically my health suffers, I don't look after myself, I eat poorly, I don't exercise, I get sick – my immune system goes, and I pick up everything from my kids. I get UTIs which turn into kidney infections, which at least means I have to rest for a few days, often after having gone to A&E for treatment.'

In the absence of a wider professional understanding of autistic burn-out in late discovered autistic women, it's our own self-knowing that is pulling us out of the trenches. Individually forensically discovering, and uncovering, episode by episode, the culmination of stressors responsible for thrusting us (with an added side of whiplash) repeatedly into that lightless place, and indeed developing the preventative strategies that we have had to apply to try and keep ourselves from falling back into the muddy, dark, soulless trenches once again.

Stressors

'Physical, mental and emotional exhaustion brought about by a cascade of factors, there are always multiple reasons, not just one thing but they pile up and crush me.'

'Usually a period of time where I have been unable to spend regular time decompressing, being on my own and generally calming down my sensory nervous system.'

'Doing too much for too long, or having a very intense social experience like a group holiday, a wedding or a work conference.'

As human beings we all experience stress – it's a pattern of psychological, biological and behavioural responses caused by stressors. However, stressors are not universally experienced, and when we look at the autistic experience of burnout, we have additional stressors that are unique to how we experience the world which immediately puts us at a disadvantage when we are talking about our exposure to stressors in everyday life, and our susceptibility when it comes to burnout.

What one person perceives as stressful will be different to the next person, and our reaction to stress is as unique as our DNA. There is no comparison. Being self-aware and understanding your own unique stressors and how stress impacts you is a crucial part of your self-knowing when it comes to rediscovering you.

When we are exposed to what we perceive to be harm, or a threat, or bombardment of our sensory, emotional and cognitive system, the result is a cluster of physiological changes which are generally referred to as our stress response. All stressors – i.e. the experiences that induce our stress response – produce a core pattern of physiological changes.

When our stress response is triggered, it activates the hypothalamus, which in turn activates our SNS (sympathetic nervous system) which then stimulates the release of the hormones adrenaline and noradrenaline from the adrenal gland into our bloodstream – often referred to as our 'fight or flight' (but there are more stress responses than just fight or flight, e.g. freeze, fawn and flop) – and when you are autistic I've concluded that there's an additional response.

It's the 'need to make it make sense' response. We are chronically misunderstood, so we've learned as a trauma response to try and make ourselves understood. Slide decks, internalized analysis from every possible angle, metaphors, over explaining, over justifying, mindmaps, scripting. All in the name of being understood by people who don't see or understand us.

Our stress response serves a catabolic function in that it mobilizes our body and brain for response and it's highly adaptive, it has evolved to enable us to deal with acute (short-lived) environmental and physical threats. During chronic stress there is frequent and prolonged activation of our nervous system which can lead to damage and disruption of our biological systems and activate the stress response on a more long-term basis; it can feel like there is no 'off switch' and the stress response becomes more damaging than the stressor itself. In psychology, we refer to this as the 'allostasis and allostatic load'.

Think of the allostatic load as overload; I imagine it as a shopping bag full to the brim of items and eventually the bottom splitting and everything spilling out on the pavement – this constant 'on' switch can have a negative impact on our health and trigger stress related illness. In fact there is a whole school of knowledge known as psychoneuroimmunology or 'PNI' for short which explores the stress vs immune system relationship, but interestingly very little research when it comes to the autistic experience, and even less to the late discovered autistic women's experience, although there is a growing body of research which suggests that there is a correlation between neurodivergence and chronic pain and illness.

Chronic stress impacts our immune system and can lead to problems in both our physical health and our cognitive health, and high levels of cortisol can lead to changes in brain function at a cellular level, we know that BDNF (brain derived neurotrophic factor) is a really important chemical in neurogenesis. Research (Kim & Kim, 2023) shows that 'chronic stress can affect our neuronal properties and cognitive functioning of the hippocampus, and at the cellular level, stress has been shown to alter hippocampal synaptic plasticity'.

Which makes me think about the levels of cortisol in autistic people when we are exposed from our very conception to unique stressors in a world that isn't built for our brains, and how that chronic stress exposure then impacts our immune system, as well as our gastrointestinal system – there's no wonder mental health conditions and chronic pain and illness are so prevalent in our community when we are in constant stress mode activation and our nervous systems are under attack.

In the 1990s there was a really important advance in our understanding of the stress response with the discovery that stressors produce physiological reactions that participate in the body's inflammatory responses. Stressors produce an increase in blood levels of cytokines – a group of peptide hormones that are released by cells in our bodies and that participate in a range of physiological and immunological responses – causing inflammation and fever.

A more recent study (Klopack *et al.*, 2022) by researchers at the University of Southern California found that stress accelerates ageing of the immune system – potentially increasing our risk of cancer, cardiovascular disease and illness from infections such as COVID-19. They found that those who were more stressed had older-seeming immune profiles – making us more susceptible to ill health.

Is there any wonder then as autistic people we are more likely to experience co-occurring chronic pain and experience ill health? I explore this in more depth over in Chapter 10.

Mitigating factors

One of the most obvious (and kindest) things we can do to prevent and mitigate burnout is to reduce our stressors – not always an easy thing to do as autistic people, as many of our stressors sit outside our control and we are often dependent on others accommodating our needs, but it's something for you to explore in terms of the stressors that you *can* control and how you self-advocate and seek out accommodations for those you cannot.

We can't simply just start refilling the shopping bag again. We have to be mindful about filling it with less things, saying no to others adding things, seeking out a bigger sturdier bag or getting help in carrying the load. Something has to fundamentally change to prevent the bottom falling out of the bag again and again. Yet asking for help is so often the thing we find hardest when we've spent a lifetime having our needs dismissed and ignored.

And even more obvious mitigating factors are our activity levels, engagement in our passions, nutritional health and sleep – all ways we can slow the damage and protect ourselves against stress related immune ageing. However, these are all things we struggle with within the autistic experience because of how we experience the world. Many in our autistic community experience co-occurring conditions that limit their ability when it comes to activity levels; many experience chronic fatigue, sensory sensitivity to food, cognitive struggles with meal planning, and struggles with sleep – again, something we will explore more in Chapter 10.

Here some of our Late Discovered Community share their experiences of how they have sought to reduce their stressors and mitigate future episodes of burnout.

'A big change I have made is changing my career. I now have control over my calendar which means I can plan in decompression time. I am also much more mindful of my social calendar and trying to have a good mix of social time and alone time.'

'As a perimenopausal working mum to teenagers with intense needs (one autistic, the other ADHD), there is always a lot to juggle! I've had to reduce my work hours from five days to three each week, and build in regular time on my own to recharge.'

'Becoming much more mindful and conscious of my behaviours, noticing when I am working too much, when I let my self-healing work slip. Incorporating self-healing work on a daily basis, and being kind to myself if I forget.'

'I've intentionally sought jobs that are more flexible, worked part-time, current role is hybrid – it's made a big difference.'

'Learning how to say NO, or just not engaging with people that will take advantage of my endless capacity to get things done, or to solve problems, or my capacity to care. I spend a lot of time at weekends talking through things with my husband to get his sense of where I'm in danger of overstretching myself or being overstretched.'

The missing link

I have had numerous periods and episodes of burnout in my life-time, and my body raises the alarm by allowing me to 'feel' the exhaustion – 'burnout throat', UTIs and ear infections are what I now understand to be my physical red flags.

However, the missing link during those episodes was the knowledge and understanding of *what* was happening and *why*. Without an understanding of autism, or the frame, nothing made sense. One of the first burnout episodes I had was when I was working as a strategist in the NHS in my early 30s. My role involved so many (now known, but then unknown) stressors that are unique to the autistic experience. I can look back now, with the knowledge I have, with a feeling of inevitability to what happened next.

Without knowing what accommodations and adaptations I needed to help prevent that episode of burnout, I found myself ultimately having to leave a role I loved and the security of paid employment, in lieu of needing to drastically change how I work because my body and nervous system couldn't cope.

Looking back now, the stressors were the combination of working in an open plan office, the daily commute to work, the office small talk, the kettle and watercooler conversations and expectations, the eating with others, the frequent train travel to London, the overnight hotel stays, the pressure to present in person without access to the scripts I now know that I need, the 'on demand' responses in meetings, the need to be social, the having to navigate my way around a city and always getting lost, struggling with reading google maps, finding the underground a sensory nightmare – all of that in parallel to blended family life, painful hips and multiple surgeries, recurrent UTIs and little to no space or solitude to decompress and sense make.

It was too much; my stress response was constantly on.

It was during one particular trip to London when my body screamed 'enough' and I experienced what felt like a panic attack as I was queueing on the tube platform ahead of a busy day of work. I couldn't get on the tube, and after a cup of tea, a biscuit and some kindness from strangers I had calmed down enough to be able to get myself on the first train back home.

My doctor diagnosed me with stress and I was signed off work for four weeks. It was during that enforced 'downtime' that I concluded that I needed to fundamentally change the way I worked, and that working for myself seemed to be the only option. That decision kickstarted a chain of events and was the point I made the scary decision to take a great leap into the unknown and to switch careers, and to follow my dream of becoming a psychotherapist. My drive was to create a compassionate space to sit in the dark with women – championing their stories and 'bringing sparkle back', and to find a better way of working that was more attuned to my needs.

And although I'd addressed many of the stressors by taking myself out of paid employment and into self-employment and a working environment I had more autonomy and control over, in the process of growing my brand and business I also created new stressors – being immersed in my passion I've discovered there is no 'off' switch. My mind is full to the brim of ideas, and it never stops, which is both a strength and a gigantic struggle, my mind eventually and inevitably crashes and my body screams enough.

My monotropic mind needs that hook of interest and attention, and working for myself there are no limitations on that constant need to create and find meaning – my mind is a buzzing hive of ideas. I become so focused (what others describe as 'drive') and all-consumed in whatever that interest is, that I eventually run out of air on my deep dive and come up to the surface almost lifeless. If you're deep diving and don't have the language or knowledge to frame that understanding then there's an added vulnerability, and inevitability for burnout – you have to be attuned to know when you are running out of air, to know when to ask for help, to know when there is danger ahead, to incorporate rest, and to know how to tune into your own frequency.

And the sad thing is that once we've hit burnout, deep diving is off the menu because we lack the energy to engage in the very things that bring us joy. I wouldn't describe my burnout as depression, but surface level living when you are in burnout feels soulless and lifeless.

There was a point at the beginning of the pandemic where I had to have an MRI scan on my brain to work out why I was struggling to talk, why I was getting my words so muddled up. Thankfully, nothing showed up on the scan and my symptoms were put down to stress. Meanwhile, my overspills and shutdowns were increasing, as was my need for solitude, verbal shutdown and the need to strategically retreat from a world that felt too much.

Sensory input across all of my senses became unbearable, my energy levels the lowest they have ever been, and I experienced more frequent UTIs and repeated ear infections than I ever have. In the space of 18 months I had over ten ear infections, and Christmas 2021 was a write off with the worst ear pain I think I've ever experienced.

I also had several covid episodes and chronic all over body pain – my body was screaming enough (again!). I can now recognize that I've been living in a perpetual state of burnout for a very long time. My body has been telling me, but I've not been dialled into the right frequency to hear that message loud and clear.

In and amongst all of this was lockdown, which helped to dial down so much of the sensory overload and gave me the space I craved to discover my hidden autistic self. An all too familiar story in our Late Discovered Community – it seems lockdown life worked better for us than any other time in our lives, the space and pace tailored to the autistic experience.

My late discovery itself was a discombobulating time because my deep dive then became the unravelling of my entire world, but it enabled me to be better attuned to knowing what I need, and importantly how to show up for myself in a way I've never known how to or why to before.

On a day-to-day level, this looked like acknowledging to myself that I didn't have the energy on the school run for small talk in the playground and giving myself permission for a self-led verbal shutdown. Or meeting a friend for dinner and explaining I couldn't sit on the table we'd been seated at, and taking us off to the quietest table in the restaurant.

I gave myself permission to make the adaptations and adjustments I need to enable me to sit on the other side of burnout. As I emerged from that unravelling, my rediscovered self was feeling depleted and exhausted from what had felt like a never-ending terrain I've had to climb, I was then presented with the Mount Everest of mountains.

The breast cancer mountain.

My life as I knew it changed in an instant.

With no other option but to climb it over the course of 18 months of treatment, the only way forwards was up. Getting to the top and planting my colourful flag before (hopefully) making my way back down the other side. Knowing that there were those who had come before me and had made it to the top, and others who had lost their lives along the climb – there were no guarantees on this mountain climb.

For the first time in my life I was faced with the confrontation of my own mortality.

I was in survival mode, and in order to prepare myself mentally for the climb of a lifetime ahead of me I was drawn to my past survival skills, the things that have got me through previous hard times – hope, determination, structure and routine, writing, relentless optimism, strength, vulnerability, courage and my beautiful, visual, creative autistic mind. In my case, I didn't get to choose my mountain, it chose me, and it's not the mountain that I will conquer on this climb but myself.

This was the universe forcing me to slow down, forcing me to reassess, forcing me to press pause, forcing me into a lockdown style hibernation, forcing me to have to live my life at a pace I've never experienced, forcing me to make my world smaller, forcing me to work in a different way, forcing me to lean into all the healing tools I've added to my toolbox over the years, forcing me to make space for myself, forcing me to see my world through yet another new vista.

And for what felt like the first time in my life I was able to ask for the space and accommodations I needed without the guilt. I had no hesitations in telling people what I needed during my cancer climb. Nobody questioned me saying no to things when I could explain the reason why and nobody placed any expectations on me other than giving me whatever space and healing time I needed. Everyone around me was flexible, supportive and adaptable to my needs. I could use my voice to advocate for my needs and accommodations. People totally get physical illness, but it shouldn't take something as extreme as cancer to realize that I can have that voice and that it's ok.

My hope?

That I emerge from this expedition with a second chance to live my life with even more self-compassion and self-knowing than when I started it, with an emboldened commitment to a more gentle, slower and meaningful life and one that is, by design, tuned into my frequency. I want to hear the beautiful music.

Burnout prevention and mitigation isn't just about making changes to how we work, it's about the changes we need to make to *how* we need to live our life. The wholesale changes that we make in our lives to honour our unique experience of the world, and it's a constant work in progress; because frequencies aren't static, we have to continually adjust and adapt to feel that sense of balance and attunement.

'Communicating that I am in burnout and cancelling all unnecessary events so that I can have the weekend/however long I can get to be completely by myself. Sleeping, engaging in favourite old special interests and taking the pressure to do anything productive completely off my shoulders really helps.'

'When I feel myself entering burnout I reinstate what I call the "bed day" rule. Basically, I take one day at the weekend and spend the whole day either in or on my bed, watching TV, reading etc.'

'Physical rest, time in solitude, not talking, reading, bingeing a TV series.'

Lowering the demands we place on ourselves.

Self-advocating.

Match funding the kindness we show in abundance to others towards ourselves.

And just as important is feeling seen, heard, understood, supported and accommodated by the people in our inner and wider world.

'It is not laziness or an inability to cope with stress, it is the result of prolonged overstimulation, which can actually often be avoided if reasonable adjustments are made.'

It's coming home to yourself – the cosy, warm place you call home.

Sit with that feeling, and imagine what that cosy, warm place you call home *could* feel like.

EXPLORING *YOUR* EXPERIENCES OF BURNOUT

By sharing our experiences of burnout in this chapter, my hope is that you have been able to learn more about stressors and triggers, and resonate with others in our community who have described what autistic burnout looks like and feels like for them, what has helped them in terms of recovery. Most importantly, I hope this has increased your understanding of the preventative measures (the changes) we make that can help us through and out of burnout.

Community as always pulls us through.

I hope that it gives you a frame to think about your own burnout experiences so that you can begin to understand and develop your own knowledge and your own autistic burnout survival guide.

- Thinking now about your own experiences, what has triggered burnout for you?

- What are your main stressors right now in your life? There is an exercise in the Frequency Circle in Chapter 12 to help you identify your stressors so that you are more aware of what they are for you.

- What does burnout feel like for you and what helps you to recover from burnout?

- What changes have you had to make and what do you recognize that helps you to prevent burnout?

And here's a whopper of a question to ponder and reflect on:

- What and how do I need my life to be?

This might be one you need to sit with and percolate for a while. Because one thing is for sure, without change we will continue to repeat the cycle of burnout.

And finally as part of your exploration, what would you like a loved one or someone in your life to know about burnout? Here's what some of our Late Discovered Community said in response to that question:

'It's not my fault and if I could do life and "normal" things without the risk of burnout, believe me I would. Burnout is serious – at its worst it makes me suicidal. I *have* to mitigate it to stay well and be the best, most productive version of myself.'

'There are many ways to offer support to an individual going through burnout and judgement is probably the worst thing one can do. There is no one single reason for burnout. It is a multitude of things that converge and completely make an individual feel like they are just drowning and not like themselves.'

CHAPTER 8

The Goldilocks Effect

Being a child of the 70s I vividly remember the story of Goldilocks and the three bears. The story of how a young girl stumbles across a cabin in the woods which is home to three bears, and whilst the bears were out on their morning walk, Goldilocks sat in each of their chairs, laid in each of their beds and ate each of their bowls of porridge until she found one that was 'just right'.

The story made me think about how Goldilocks clearly had sensory sensitivities and needed her immediate world to feel 'just right' – from the temperature of the porridge to the comfiness of the bed – and how she was framed as 'fussy' and 'demanding'. And maybe this fairytale struck me as an undiscovered autistic child because Goldilocks was showing me the inside story into her world, that would have also looked like my world. Maybe reading it as a child I absorbed how Goldilocks was framed as being 'fussy' and 'demanding' – her needs were 'too much'.

I'll never really know, but as I embarked on my own late discovery journey and into this new world that I would come to call home, the story of Goldilocks and the three bears came back to me, because when you've spent a lifetime being told that you are too much, seen as fussy, demanding, difficult, intense, selfish, controlling and inflexible because you need 'everything just right' in your environment to function, or you've been harmed, bullied, marginalized or humiliated by others because of who you are, how do you begin to lower that mask when your needs conflict with others?

When we mask, we effectively put others' needs before our own, scared to ask for what we need in case we're seen as different, or given the Goldilocks label, so we take the long way round or we endure pain and discomfort because we live in fear of what might happen to us, or how unlovable we might be. We consistently override our inner warning system. Is there any wonder burnout then becomes inevitable? It's our body saying it can't take anymore, and masking is not easy to unpick when it's been your default for so long.

Recent research (Pearson & Rose, 2023) defines autistic masking as:

> a form of identity management involving consciously or unconsciously suppressing aspects of identity and action. Often seen in socially marginalised groups, it is found to contribute towards poorer outcomes for autistic people and is related to higher prevalence of suicidality, exhaustion, burnout, and mental health difficulties.

In their extensive work on this subject they suggest that there is often a misconception and that there has been a long-standing belief that autistic masking is a social strategy. This implies that it's some conscious choice we have made and that in any given situation we can then choose not to mask, which underpins this myth that exists about masking being a manipulative tool that we can pick up and put down at any point we choose.

However, what we know from emerging research that has been undertaken and co-produced with autistic people, as well as from the many stories and experiences we hear in our Late Discovered Club Community, is that masking is rooted in trauma. It's a safety mechanism, a survival skill that we have to learn so early in our lives, borne out of the stigma and invalidation we have all experienced. We use it to keep ourselves safe, to self-protect and to fit in more. We learn very early on that who we are is not how others want us to be. Every aspect of our autistic selves is invalidated from a very young age. We mask to self-protect and to create psychological safety in a world that feels unsafe (Pearson & Rose 2023).

And as we navigate our own late discovery and begin to understand our own individual needs it can often feel like we become 'more autistic' when actually it was there all along. Masking can look like being the 'quiet' or 'shy' one, the 'funny' one, the people pleaser or, conversely, an exaggerated version of ourselves – we feed the confirmation bias of what we think others want or expect to see, and it becomes a heavy survival mechanism to maintain.

And we don't just mask, we mirror, we compensate, we accommodate and we camouflage – the art of blending ourselves into our environments – how we talk, how we act, how we show up, how we dress. We compensate too through scripting and learning social rules and cues, and looking at how others do it, and we assimilate by putting on an act, or we need others to support us when we are socializing.

What I've seen in my work with now several hundred late discovered autistic women is that we are more likely to mirror and mask, just as we are more likely to withdraw than act out, and have more 'socially acceptable' interests, which is in part why we manage to go under the radar for so long and remain undiscovered, but we know that the fallout from a lifetime of masking is related to higher prevalence of suicidality, exhaustion, burnout and mental health difficulties.

And if you are a late discovered woman who is black or brown, and/or gender non-conforming, and/or from the LGBTQIA+ community then masking and the associated fallout becomes even more prevalent due to the additional layers of discrimination and stigmatization associated with these intersecting identities.

Laid bare

I spent the first four decades of my life never really verbalizing my struggles or differences because I was unaware of what they were exactly, suppressing, and feeling like I didn't belong. Living my life behind a mask watching everyone else who seemed to meander through life immune to the struggles I was experiencing.

I can recognize now that I developed many compensation

strategies to help me out in situations I struggled in, especially social situations. I would always try to be the organizer and the person making sure everyone else is ok, that way the spotlight is off me. I'd surround myself with people who are the life and soul and enjoy being centre stage – my very own social aid. I'd ask lots of questions and be curious of others, and try to maintain the expected eye contact and the right amount of facial expressions, yet underneath it I'd be feeling unnaturally forced. I'd always look immaculate and dress in clothes that stand out so that the conversation and gaze is always about what I'm wearing as opposed to what I'm doing (or not).

I always had an exit strategy from any event – sit at the back, look busy and always have a time limit on how long I'd stay and a long list of excuses as to why I had to leave or give my apologies. I'd use alcohol for the social armour if it was an enforced event. I'd be figuring out what people are *really* thinking by being tuned into their facial expressions, body language and tone of voice. And the thing with compensation strategies is that they don't always work or go to plan; they are also exhausting.

And every time I responded with overwhelm or burnout or shutdown, or found myself overspilling with emotion and tears, or bed bound with a UTI or ear infection, it deepened the shame that I felt about myself. When we have to mask it reinforces a message that who we are is not acceptable or palatable, and it's a draining and depleting way to live your life, it means your *whole* self is never really on full show or fully embraced.

I'm aware that, by writing this book, what lies beneath that mask is being laid bare, and there's something hugely liberating and freeing about not just showing the world who I am, but giving myself the permission to embrace my differences – to no longer feel the darkness of shame.

'Fifteen months on after my self-discovery I am unmasking in my own presence. My mind is no longer filled with thoughts and trains of thoughts swirling off about the why, hows and ifs of my behaviours alone or out in the world. I know now why my brain is as it is and no longer have to try and work it out. So there is no mask for me with myself.

With others it is a work in progress. With a few, mainly new, friends I do not mask at all. I say what is on my mind, say why I can or cannot do a particular activity, e.g. be in a large group, go to a party. And we work something out or put it into a maybe in the future place.

Sometimes I catch myself masking. I am really interested and curious about people, but struggle with a two-way continuing, connected conversation. I find myself slipping back into asking questions repeatedly and I think stop, take a pause, go with the flow.'

'Learning about my mask has freed me from it. It was heavy and I'm glad I don't have to carry it constantly anymore. I have now quite publicly self-disclosed which I feel will help me in allowing myself to just be myself.'

Spaces, faces and places

However, I'm also acutely aware that I live sandwiched between my authentic autistic self and the neuronormative standards and views that dominate the world in which we live and that if we are going to mask less, then we need psychologically safe spaces, faces and places to unmask.

I know that there will always be spaces, faces and places that aren't safe for me to be my whole autistic self in or around. The reality is that we have to curate our own that feel 'just right', but to do that we have to have choice, autonomy and the self-knowing and self-permission to design the frequency we want and need (and deserve) to listen to. We also need allies, supporters and champions who will make it their mission to understand us, accommodate us, love us and celebrate us for our differences.

Only the other day I was having coffee with a friend and we were talking about the progress of this book. I was telling her how much I had written in the space of a cold week of hibernation in January, and she responded with how that was down to the power of my beautiful autistic brain. She is someone I can be my whole self with, someone I don't have to use those compensation strategies with, which makes social interaction with this person feel lighter, and without the need for decompression afterwards.

It's something I am aware of when I'm in the company of other autistic people, creating a neuro-inclusive environment for them to be able to show up without the masking, whether that's in a post discovery support circle or interviewing a guest on the podcast, I will set the scene by saying that it doesn't matter about eye contact, or whether you are using a script, or whether you want your camera off. In the circles, we offer the option to participate by writing in the chat function if a person's capacity is low that day and their speech is not fluid as a result, and in doing that, I imagine if someone created that space for me, how freeing and safe that would feel.

We all need more of that, but if you're not autistic you'll be oblivious to what is happening on the inside and how it feels to be in those situations. We are the ones given the stereotype about 'lacking empathy' but what I see is that empathy is a two-way street – what we call the double empathy problem (also known as the double empathy gap) – something I talk about more in the next chapter.

Post discovery, that new, clearer view out of the window means masking becomes a much more conscious process, but the reality is that we are so far from a society that is accommodating or understanding, and conscious masking is exhausting – it's a constant environmental safety scan.

- Considering what the impact might be?

- Will I be treated differently?

- Will I be harmed?

- What will happen to me?

Sometimes we are forced into unmasking because we are in distress, or because we need accommodations from others. However, what I've learned from experience is that unmasking can cause even more distress and harm if the person we unmask to invalidates or doesn't see us, or responds in a way that makes us feel like we are being difficult, or assumes we lack competency and talks to us like we are a child, because their understanding of autism is lacking.

Their mountain top

I've found some situations immediately made me feel dehumanized and 'othered' when I disclosed and unmasked myself, but I am now more able to reframe them, and stand on *their mountain top* and see some truths in those situations and this is what I see:

- They don't have any understanding of what autism is – that's on them not me.

- It's not my job to educate them, it's for them to do the work.

- I am not going to allow them to hold that amount of power over me.

- Their opinion of me doesn't make me any less.

- I have no control over anyone else's responses other than my own.

I disclosed my autism as I started on the breast cancer mountain climb to the team who were responsible for my care, and shared the accommodations that I would need. As I progressed on my climb and I met with different health professionals along the way, how I was treated varied. There was one health professional, who spoke to me like a child, who assumed that I didn't understand what she was telling me, and also assumed that my adult daughter who came along to the appointment with me was my 'carer'.

Then there was the one who said to me that I didn't look autistic because I was so articulate in the written complaint that I had made during one traumatic acute hospital stay where my needs weren't accommodated or listened to. Another who assumed that my over-spill and eventual shutdown during a hospital stay was because I was scared of being in hospital. I wasn't scared, I was in sensory and pain overload. Yet this health professional came to their own conclusion about my experience without actually asking me.

It was clear to me that unmasking wasn't safe for me in the hospital environment that I found myself immersed in, I feared what would happen to me on future acute stays and I felt othered and misunderstood, which led me to transferring my care part way through my treatment to a hospital further away from home which added extra travel time and costs but was the right decision for me to access the care I needed.

I was given the opportunity to speak to the consultant oncologist who would be responsible for my care and explain what I needed and why. It was also a specialist cancer centre, the largest in Europe, and I instantly felt safer by the interactions I had with the professionals who were involved in my care. And I have no doubt that reducing stress during 18 months of cancer treatment will be a key contributor to the outcome of my cancer recovery and survivorship.

Language and understanding is power

We underestimate how fundamental language is when we are safety scanning spaces, faces and places. I can tell how much someone understands autism by the language they use, and if it's patholo-gizing and non-affirming then it's code to me that this is not a safe place for me to be in, or to reveal my autistic self. Since my discov-ery, masking has become more of a conscious process, and I have worked hard on creating safe spaces, faces and places where I can be my whole self, and my world is now majority unmasked – work, home, my parents, and my closest friendships, I can show up as my whole self, unleashing my autistic joy. I can only imagine what peace that now brings to my nervous system.

My home, which I share with my neurodivergent children, is a low demand, environmentally sound, sensory friendly and neuro compassionate space. Individually we have distinct struggles, support needs and strengths and we are attuned and supportive of each other. We openly stim, are all appreciative of how important space, solitude and decompression time is to retune our nervous system and we recognize how meaningful and vital it is that our monotropic minds have the opportunity to deep dive into whatever interest or passion we are consumed by and finding joy in.

Different forms of communication are welcome and respected depending on current capacity and overload, and our downtime is 'downtime' not filled with the things that disrupt our frequency. And my seven-year-old has known the language of 'spoons' since she was little – she knows what depletes them and what replenishes them, and she's able to verbalize and articulate her needs more and more, which gives her autonomy in her own frequency balance.

Spoon theory has nothing to do with eating, but everything to do with energy – *your* energy – on a day-to-day basis. It comes from the idea that if you are living with chronic pain, illness or any condition that causes fatigue then you have less energy on a day-to-day basis to do even the basic everyday tasks.

Imagine each day you wake with a certain number of spoons and that each spoon equals a unit of energy – straightaway you could be in a deficit because you've not slept well or you are in pain. Spoons vary based on demands and activities, and some days they are so depleted. Rather than continuing to do things that continue to deplete them, or see you borrowing spoons, your focus has to shift to spoon recovery and replenishment.

We talk in the currency of spoons in our multiply neurodivergent house, and 'not having enough spoons' or 'I don't have the spoons to do that today' or 'I only have enough spoons to do one thing today' are phrases we use all too often, and the solution is low demand living.

I'm always amazed by what other people who don't experience energy as a rare precious resource manage to pack in on evenings and weekends, and how we compare ourselves and all the 'shoulds' and guilt we carry.

What does low demand look like for me?

- Using weekends, evenings and time off to decompress, recalibrate and not feeling guilty for doing so.

- Slow weekends.

- Reducing known sensory stressors.

- Removing the 'shoulds'.

- Having the autonomy and self-permission to say no to things.

- Quieter talking, the opportunity to not have to talk, communicate in other ways.

- Being aware of your current energy and capacity and matching it to your output.

- Carving out the space and solitude that you need.

- Spending your time in the places and spaces that tune into your frequency (your sensory moderators and self-connectors) which form part of my Frequency Circle in Chapter 12.

Code word

We have a safe word for when we are in social situations and it's becoming too much. Our specific code word means 'get me out of here' without having to explain why or using energy to communicate. It's code for me as her parent to say our goodbyes and retreat back to the safe and calm sanctuary of home. And I've since created a code word for myself too, for me to give myself the permission I need to 'get me out of here'.

None of this is rocket science – creating safe spaces, inclusion, acceptance and belonging starts in our homes. It's in the language we use and the accommodations we make. It's in the love we give and the acceptance we show.

The safety scan

'I can only unmask where I feel safe, with individuals that I trust and with whom I feel safe, and this is not the case everywhere. And even if I am unmasking in public in spaces like at my workplace, I haven't told anyone (with the exception of two colleagues whom I consider friends) why I am now suddenly doing certain things or not doing others anymore. I'm just doing it without further explanations and no questions have been raised so far.'

'However, while travelling, especially as a solo, racialized female traveller, if I don't try to force some sort of eye contact or fake smiles and facial expressions, do small talk, etc. as I would very much prefer, I could find myself in a very unsafe situation very quickly. Recently I also noticed that I still feel like I have to mask in job interviews. It just doesn't feel safe to unmask and risk not making it through the process because of stigma.'

'Feeling safe. It's dependent on who I am with – I don't feel I can with all family members as they have made it very clear their views on autism, i.e. 'everyone's a little bit autistic'. Masking is exhausting, and it doesn't always feel safe to unmask, but as I've been open and honest at work, and have put adjustments in place, I've managed to work nearly full-time hours for 18 months without becoming unwell (well, only two UTIs, but no hospital).'

However, there are still spaces, faces and places unfortunately where the need to mask remains for me, and my safety scan is on the lookout for any red flags:

- Judgement
- Bias

- Lacking in understanding and compassion

- Language

- Body language

- Past history – what's in the evidence bank? Being trauma informed. Have I been harmed by this place, space or face in the past? What associations have I attached to them?

If I'm having to put myself into a situation where I'm going to compromise my own needs for others, there are a number of questions I now have to ask myself and consider whether it's something I want to do, and if I choose not to, be comfortable with facing whatever consequences arise.

- Q. What will it take from me?

- Q. What's the cost? Emotionally, physically, psychologically?

- Q. Do I have the spoons/capacity?

- Q. What do I need to do for myself to accommodate it?

- Q. What boundaries do I need to self-impose?

- Q. How can I protect myself?!

- Q. What adaptations can I make to lessen the impact on my nervous system?

- Q. Is the juice worth the squeeze?

The safety scan looks like being much more aware of my needs, anticipating situations and triggers, giving myself permission to do what is needed, making accommodations for myself, and ultimately being kinder and more compassionate towards myself.

However, sometimes the safety scan doesn't have time to come into play. Sometimes we find ourselves in situations where self-disclosure happens without being able to risk assess the potential fallout. The advocacy role we find ourselves having to take on without choice in situations is exhausting. As well as the unmasked stigmatizing hangover we feel with people who really don't understand us, and the subsequent feeling you then get of being forever 'observed' after you've been put into an unsafe situation of self-disclosure.

For so many autistic people their worlds, homes, families and workplaces are not a safe place to be themselves. We need and deserve to live in a world which is filled with more autistic allies in all our spaces and places.

Find your allies. They will be the people who make you feel safe, regulated and accepted. Not observed, not tolerated, not too much and not too demanding. There is no place in your rediscovered world for those faces, spaces and places who scramble your frequency.

Coming home means giving yourself permission to design a world for yourself that is underpinned by your own self-knowing and your own self-needs, and that looks different for us all because we are all different, and all at different starting points.

Remind yourself that you are allowed to create spaces and places that feel safe and nourishing.

This is your rediscovered world.

> 'Sometimes I do not care and I am me, predominantly in my safe places of somatic movement and dance and with the people I know through these circles. Not with others who I perceive as being critical of my way of being. Sometimes cautious, a dipping my toe in approach to see what happens, to continue or retreat.'

> 'Stimming has been revealed as my mask lifts, which has been quite amazing. I recognized a joy in stimming in dance, figure of eight movements through my hips and spine, seeing what movement emerges. Joyous and fun.'

'With my family (parents mainly), I've not fully shared my diagnosis, and with my mother particularly, I don't feel like I could share or unmask – she finds me hard enough to interact with in full masking mode, it would be game over if I was unmasked and fully me with her. With my dad, I suspect he's on the spectrum too, and he and I have always been very similar, so I feel like I can unmask quite a bit with him.'

'I now openly tell people that I will not come to big social gatherings/events because I do not feel comfortable or I simply do not want to – without inventing silly excuses that made it sound like I really wanted to be there but I can't. The truth is I do not want to be there. And even if I don't say it openly to others, just acknowledging it for myself, is an expression of unmasking for me.'

'I am also now giving myself much more freedom around echolalia. I used to repeat things such as key words, license plate numbers, codes, constantly only in my mind and now I am repeating them out loud and it gives me a lot of comfort.'

'I am still trying to work out where my "mask" starts and where I begin. I find it very difficult to work out when I am actually masking most of the time. I think I have leaned into my instincts to stim more, especially when it comes to fidgeting and dancing to music. I bring blu tac with me to meetings and when travelling to play with, and I listen to music and dance while I do chores at home.'

'I'm being much more open with my family about my feelings and my needs. I'm learning to say when I need some time out to be on my own.'

 EXPLORING *YOUR* EXPERIENCES OF MASKING

Give yourself some time and space in this chapter to self-reflect and think about your own masking story as you read through the experiences of other late discovered women from our community.

There's often a misconception that masking and the associated 'unmasking' is about taking off 'a mask'. The reality is that there are multiple layers to this mask, and it's a day to day, situation to situation, person to person, experience sensitive approach to peeling back the multifaceted layers. Becoming more aware is really the big first step.

- Is masking something that you recognize you do? What are the places, spaces and faces where you have to mask? And why?

It might be that, even despite not knowing you were autistic growing up, you had caregivers who you didn't have to mask around and that in your home environment you were largely unmasked and accommodated. Conversely you may have had the complete opposite.

- Thinking back to growing up, was it safe for you to be yourself?

- As you're navigating this brave new rediscovered world, have you recognized that you've begun to peel back some of those layers?

- Does it feel safe for you to unmask? At home? With your family? At work? Amongst friends?

- What helps you to be more you? What are the places, spaces and faces where you can be you?

- What do you recognize you need to do more of or less of in this brave new rediscovered world?

- What do you need from others to help you peel back those layers of your mask?

CHAPTER 9

Our Social and Relational World

*Content warning: In this chapter I talk about sexual abuse and victimization.

There's a common myth and stereotype about the autistic experience that we're not sociable beings. In fact if you have been through an autism assessment which aligns itself to the current DSM-5 diagnostic criteria, you will know that we are assessed on our 'problems' and 'deficits' with our social communication and how we relate to others. The problem with this belief is that it positions us as being 'less than' – we are pathologized for our differences in how we communicate and how we relate to others.

When it comes to the autistic social and relational world, we may communicate differently to the neuronormative and our relational expectations may look different too, but that doesn't mean we're not social beings, that we don't need or seek out connection. The difference is that we seek it out in ways that are meaningful to how we each individually experience the world.

As autistic people we feel the world and our emotions more deeply, and have neurons that are always on and firing. Our sensory and nervous system experiences the world more intensely, and we have to process more incoming data – it's a lot. There's no wonder then that we may need our own language to navigate our social and relational worlds or that we might seek to meet our social and relational needs in a way that supports our own world view, and as a consequence our communication styles will differ from the neuronormative.

And when we find others who can communicate and understand our language it tunes us into our frequency. There's safety, understanding and compassion present. Those who understand, for example, that spoken word shutdown is not a euphemism for being rude but rather a safety mechanism when there's too much input and we may need to communicate in other ways.

Or those who don't insist on small talk. Its surface level nature means that it doesn't serve my deep diving interest-based system. I'm often in awe of people who can swim so casually on the surface and talk about things that have no depth. Some people make surface swimming look so effortless and elegant, yet my brain does not want to engage.

I'm here for the depth.

I want and need people in my world whom I can deep dive with on a one-to-one level, who are connected to my interests. I want deep and meaningful relationships and quickly become drained in my social interactions if communication is surface level or where there is no 'in' point or hook to ever deep dive together. It's why being a podcast host and a therapist plays to my social and relational strengths – I get to dive deep.

And this is why communication in our post discovery group support circles flows so easily.

I am deeply connected to people and their stories, but I also require and need a significant amount of alone time, space and solitude where there are no demands on me to speak, and where instead I can engage in solo activities such as writing – blank pages are where I can express myself most clearly, which is why scripting works as a safety anchor for me.

There are no demands on the page, my language flows, and I can share with the world, or shield from the world within the safety of my journal. Don't assume my silence, spoken word shutdown, on demand struggle, or lack of small talk means that I have nothing to say – I have so much that I want to say, but I need to express it in a way that is meaningful for me. A silent retreat I recently attended with no demands on me to speak mouth words for three whole days was everything I needed, that I never knew I needed.

I watch TV and scroll social media with the addition of subtitles because I find it difficult to listen to something focusing solely on my hearing sense, especially when there is any other noise present. Adding in words helps me to concentrate and focus on what I'm watching. And I have also observed in myself that I enjoy talking with plenty of hand movement, but that in many situations I force myself to not gesticulate, and that I will clench my hands so tightly or will hold onto objects to prevent me from hand talking.

Since my discovery I have given myself the permission more and more to go into spoken word shutdown whenever I need to – there are so many situations where talking with the spoken word feels too much. I never really recognized or appreciated how much I needed that self-accommodation. And I'm enabling and unleashing the gesticulating whenever and however I need and want to.

Rediscovery and coming home to ourselves means being more accommodating of our needs and creating that space and solitude that we need in the ways that we need it – tuning into *our frequency*.

'I struggle to be interested in something which holds no interest for me, whether this be people, places, events. I shut off, stop listening, walk away or do not enter the situation in the first place. I guess I have been perceived as rude, and I struggle with how difficult, and at times impossible it is to engage with another person when I have lost the thread in a conversation, particularly if with more than one person.'

'I need to script social situations and check I'm not over-talking about a special interest or oversharing. My husband is my safe person and trusted adult – he's ADHD so he can talk to anyone! I hate the phone, and my preferred forms of communication are written. I find social situations are uncomfortable and require a lot of effort with people I don't know or venues I'm not familiar with.'

Sex and the City

As a 40-something woman, *Sex and the City* sold me a fantasy through my TV screen in so many ways. From the stilettos to the style, but on a much deeper level too it propagated a female friendship myth that left me feeling out of the picture. *Sex and the City's* worldview suggests that we have somehow failed in life if we don't have a group of close girlfriends with whom we've grown up from infant school and meet up weekly for brunch and small talk in a busy cafe or bar.

It always intrigued me how Carrie, Miranda, Samantha and Charlotte managed to physically and mentally come together as often as they did, in between high-flying careers, relationships, kids and life generally. I would sit and watch SATC trying to figure out how they had the energy to socialize in the way that they did, and why they made it look effortless, and question why I found that hard, and why my relational needs differed.

- Why do I struggle to do more than one thing in a day (work included)?

- Why do I find school pick up and drop off so uncomfortable?

- Why do I constantly seek out places and spaces with few people?

- Why do I need so much alone time?

- Why don't I like people coming over to my house?

- Why don't I like socializing in big groups?

- Why do I prefer my socializing to be done whilst 'doing an activity'?

- Why do I need start and end times and an exit strategy?

- Why do I want to avoid family get-togethers?

- Why do I find socializing so draining?

- Why don't I need the level of interaction I see others need?

- Why was lockdown during the pandemic so liberating for me?

- Why don't I get jokes or understand sarcasm?

- Why have I experienced so much social trauma and harm in my life?

I am a sociable person, but I find socializing in the neuronormative sense hard, and recognize that I need a whole heap of alone time to prepare and recover, along with clear start and end points. Online socializing gets me round this – the voice notes back and forth with my neurodivergent friends keeps me connected. Voice notes give me the floor to speak and the time and space to listen and process, and my brain appreciates the fact that voice notes are not 'on demand'.

I have a whole constellation of friends that I have connected with over the years who aren't necessarily in the same solar system as each other, but with whom I can develop one to one relationships in a way that is meaningful for us both, but equally it's exhausting keeping up with the nurture and maintenance that all those individual people in my life need and deserve. Neurodivergent friendships are so much easier because we learn to speak each other's language, there's a deep level of understanding and seeking to understand which happens behind the scenes, rather than judgement and a whole lot more room to accommodate individual needs and preferences.

Coming home to myself was about understanding what my relational and communication needs are, accepting myself and my needs, and extending that compassion and empathy that my pre-discovered self was missing.

'I experience my friendships very intensely from an emotional standpoint, and often view them as just as important as familial and romantic relationships. I can become very overwhelmed when I feel I have upset someone, and constantly worry that I have.'

'My friends provide a lot of reassurance for me. I struggle to keep up with birthdays and regular social events or even regular communication. I am lucky that my friends understand that is not a reflection of my feelings about them.'

The double empathy problem

This 'deficit' has always landed at the feet of autistic people, but what if the problem also lies with the non-autistic people who are unable to extend empathy and understanding to our communication and relational styles because they don't look and sound like their normal?

The double empathy problem (Milton, 2012) is a theory that Dr Damien Milton, an autistic academic, came up with more than a decade ago to explain this. Simply put, his theory argues that just because autistic people experience the world differently, and interact with others and sense the world differently, it doesn't mean that we don't have emotions or feel empathy.

What Milton's theory recognizes is that these differences can make it difficult for non-autistic people to understand and empathize with autistic people and vice versa.

A double empathy problem.

However, not only are autistic people misunderstood, we're then also pathologized for our differences.

I try to liken the double empathy problem to different languages. Imagine being on holiday somewhere and you don't speak the local language. You go out for dinner and make no attempt to order your food using the language written on the menu or the language spoken by the server.

You expect the server to speak your language.

Being the server in that restaurant is what it feels like to be autistic communicating with someone who is non-autistic. I've spent a lifetime putting myself on other people's mountain tops, standing up for injustices, constantly worrying I've got something wrong or upset someone.

When you don't understand the 'rules' you do everything you can to get those rules 'right' (in the neuronormative, acceptable way) and when we get it wrong, it hits so hard. Stacked underneath the latest thing are a whole load of times we've been shamed for not getting it 'right' – the internalized shame getting bigger each and every time.

It's like we speak a whole different language. I've spent a lifetime making the effort to learn neuronormative language, and I am multilingual and can language switch (i.e. mask) at great personal expense. But those who are monolingual, who only have one language and can't or won't learn the language of autistic people, are forever going to have a view of autistic communication as problematic and less than, or a language that is too 'difficult' or 'complex' to bother learning.

It's a very ableist, highly judgemental and one-dimensional perspective which sounds like 'If you don't socialize, communicate or relate in the way that I do then there's something wrong with you and you are less than'.

What helps to close the double empathy problem is a meeting somewhere in the middle – you try to speak a bit of my language and I'll try and speak a bit of yours. Or even better, you learn my language so that you can be bi-lingual too. The only way to do that is to understand my inner world, and importantly, want to understand it.

'I am a very sporadic and transactional communicator. I find myself overwhelmed by communication demands now, the number and pervasiveness of messaging platforms. I feel like I have to read them the whole time, and then I feel pressure to immediately respond...which I don't and then it gets embarrassing about how long I've gone without responding.

I find it really stressful. Probably more stressful than actual in person interactions now. The expectation to always be available is awful and something I really struggle with.'

Safety anchors

Many autistic people have 'safe people' who are our safety anchors in life, who not only understand our language and can speak our language, but they can translate too. Our safety anchors are our safety aids, and our co-regulators. Our calm in the storm, and when we lose them through bereavement, loss and relationship break-down, it's not just the person we lose, we can become anchorless, drifting at sea.

I'm not sure that non-autistic people really comprehend the existential loss of a safety anchor. We typically give that grace of a 'grieving period' when we lose a loved one, but this is more than that. This is being alone at sea. It's no wonder then that autistic people are more likely to report experiencing PTSD related to loss and bereavement, and are vulnerable to mental health crisis and suicidality around the time of loss.

Inclusion and safety starts at home

Late autistic discovery signals change, because the more you under-stand about yourself and your needs, the less you are able to mask your needs, and what I see in our community is that our discovery can both strengthen our relationships with others *and* create con-flicts in our social and relational worlds.

Things we were perhaps tolerant of previously become impos-sible to tolerate when you have this new perspective and self-understanding. We begin to verbalize our needs more, perhaps request accommodations more, and assume our new identity, and unfortunately it's not always met with acceptance. We've been deep diving and skimming the ocean floor collecting all of this knowledge and understanding about ourselves, and yet the people around us so often just don't get it, or don't respond in the way we hoped or don't prioritize the need to learn our language.

At the point of this profound discovery, we might hear how diffi-cult we are being, questions of why can't we go back to how we were, we might see non-action at our requests for accommodations, or body language and behaviour that is code for you are asking too much. And when you have spent a lifetime not expressing your needs to be met with this, it can power up a deep sense of resentment.

What we want and need to hear

- I love you.

- I love that you now have this deep found insight and knowledge.

- I love you even more and accept you for who you are.

- What do you need?

- How can I help you?

- What can I do to try and understand you more?

- What would help make you feel safe and regulated?

- Can you help me to understand your language?

There's also the sense that continuing to live like this with this new-found knowledge will either 'break me or break us', and whilst there shouldn't have to be a choice, there often is a hard choice to be made in coming home to yourself, which is why relationship breakdown and divorce is so prevalent in our Late Discovered Community.

And whilst that's not the experience or story for all late discovered women, it is unfortunately the experience and reality for some. The dawning realization of the conflicts and so often the harm we face in our relationships. Relational advice and advocacy around coercive control, domestic abuse, support at the point of relationship breakdown, as well as navigating the divorce process is something that is missing for our community.

We need to do more.

Being an ally

> 'It's highly likely that my parents are neurodivergent, although undiagnosed. My niece is neurodivergent and my sister is wanting to explore. Neurodivergence is also present with my paternal family, but it's very much seen as a disorder, something to hide and not admit – which makes life a challenge due to the lack of acceptance of any difference and therefore they are not prepared to make or recognize accommodations needed. We have needed to distance ourselves to manage the unhelpful impact on our family.'

Autistic inclusion and affirming acceptance starts at home and in the spaces we frequent – our workplaces and our friendships. It starts with the language people use – everyone has the power to use affirming and inclusive language, to self-educate and to respect and value difference.

When we find ourselves in relational spaces post discovery where we are misunderstood, treated as being 'less than' and where difference is not embraced, it creates a relational divide and can deepen feelings of not belonging and of rejection – those cumulative layers of relational, social and interpersonal trauma are once again triggered. It's no wonder that our post-discovery world for many feels like grief work. It's loss and it's all the letting go of the people who *can't and won't* meet us where we are at.

A good place to start is in the language that you use towards yourself and that loved ones use, and this is something you can lead when it comes to the language to describe yourself. There is no right or wrong, whether it's identity first (I am autistic) or whether it's person first (I have autism), it is *your* individual choice. And you can ask your loved ones to drop the 'D's – the deficits and the disorder language, because autism is not a dirty or shameful word, it's a word that means difference. And we can celebrate difference and be accommodating of difference.

'You don't need to treat me differently now I have a diagnosis. You don't need to stop making eye contact with me in case it makes me uncomfortable (I can do that all by myself thank you). You don't need to commiserate or console me. Celebrate with me, ask me if I need any accommodations, other than that change nothing.'

Autistic women experience high rates of abuse

As a community, many of us have experienced coercive, physical or sexual abuse, yet there is a distinct lack of research out there which explores the multitude of abuse experienced by autistic women and girls.

However, a recent study in France (Cazalis *et al.*, 2022) found that nine out of ten autistic women are sexually victimized, and that whilst sexual violence affects about 30 per cent of women in the general population it is between *two to three times* as much for autistic women and at huge costs for their mental and physical health.

I was shocked, but sadly not surprised by the findings from this study. The team who undertook this research also undertook a systematic review of sexual victimization in the autistic population and concluded that 'being autistic means undergoing a 10–16% risk of enduring sexual molestation as a child and a 62–70% risk of being sexually victimised in adulthood and that most victims are girls and women'.

When they asked participants about prevention factors:

- 22% of the participants in the study said that sexual manipulators or predators seem to spot you more easily because of your difficulties in sexual interactions

- 17% said that knowledge of self-affirmation strategies learned in therapy (or social skills groups) could have helped them stay safe better

- 16% said their family members should have been more attentive

- 10% said that female teenagers and their parents should be better informed about the risk of sexual abuse

- 10% said nothing could have protected them

- 8% said that health professionals should have given adapted prevention advice such as better identifying sexually ambiguous situations with men

- 4% said that the officials of the institution (high school, university, company) in which they were should have been more watchful.

The authors of the study say:

> that it would be a methodological and deontological mistake to consider that victimisation in autistic women is mainly due to autism. On the contrary, we postulate that the main cause of sexual violence against autistic women is their womanhood, since perpetrators preferably target women and girls. Therefore, it is reasonable to consider that autism is *not the cause* of sexual victimisation in autistic women but a factor increasing their vulnerability.

And whilst the researchers suggest that autism is not the cause, but an additional factor, it doesn't negate the very real fact that so many late discovered autistic women have found themselves over the span of many decades in relationships, friendships, situations, families and workplaces which are trauma inducing, abusive, coercive or controlling. They have been repeatedly bullied, ghosted and marginalized. The social and relational trauma all adds up.

The vulnerability factor is perhaps that you believe that people have good intentions (like you) and you have a strong ethical and moral compass (doesn't everyone?). Added to this, you are a chronic under-placer of your own needs, never want to get anything wrong, experience differences in communication and emotional processing, and your self-esteem has never had the opportunity to bloom.

Add in over-giving and under-receiving, a propensity to go into spoken word shutdown or complete freeze response when faced with situations that are harmful to you, or conversely 'flighting' but finding yourself stuck and unable to leave the situation you are in, a lifetime of being gaslit about what you are experiencing and feeling, on top of not actually knowing that you are autistic – people take advantage and cause harm.

However, let's be very clear here that the fault and responsibility sits firmly with the person inflicting the harm and abuse. Your gender and your neurotype does not mean that you are responsible for, nor deserving of, the harm that you have suffered. The blame lies entirely with the perpetrator.

The authors of the study go on to say that:

Prevention is absolutely necessary, certainly not in the sole form of sex education but rather by promoting profound cultural changes such as recommended by the Center for Disease Control (CDC) and World Health Organization (WHO): both organizations indeed strongly affirm that the very root of sexual violence is gender inequality.

And the reality is that even when we do speak up and speak out about the harm that we have experienced, it's all too often dismissed, gaslit, not believed, or it's our autism that's 'to blame'.

Perpetrators of abuse are everywhere, they walk amongst us, and are less likely to be random strangers; rather they are the people in our everyday lives, people we trust and people who are 'trusted' by others.

If you want to be an ally and protect the next generation of autistic girls and women from harm, then you need to be aware and understand the increased risk factors and take action to safeguard them.

Being autistic and experiencing sexual victimization should not be two things that inevitably go together just because of your gender and your neurotype.

Where is the outrage?

Where is the protection and safeguarding?

Where is the understanding and the allyship?

We deserve more.

Interpersonal victimization

The victimization of autistic people by familiar others (interpersonal victimization) is all too present in the experiences of our Late Discovered Club Community, yet it's an understudied phenomenon, and again there is very little to no research specifically when it comes to autistic women and how they experience interpersonal victimization.

Another recent study (Pearson *et al.*, 2022) found that:

autistic adults experience victimisation from a range of close others, and may find it difficult to recognise when someone is acting in an abusive manner. Many participants had experienced heightened compliance in response to unreasonable requests from others, however, reasons for this were varied (e.g. fear, desire to avoid confrontation) and require further investigation.

Furthermore 'these findings have implications for developing supports which enable autistic adults to recognise their own boundaries and advocate for themselves, in addition to helping them to recognise what a healthy relationship looks like'.

'According to my sister I've always been vulnerable and picked friends that need me for something and who take advantage of me. And she's right. It's only now that I'm older that I've realized that I don't actually need many friends.'

'I have one amazing close friend who I've known for 20 years and is so supportive of me. But I've been used, blown out, ignored, dropped out of groups. I've never understood why, I always just thought it was because I was too much hard work.'

'I have always thought that my personality made me prone to abuse by others. I have experienced it firsthand in a workplace setting whereby my autistic traits made it easier for someone else to abuse their power and made an unbearable working environment for myself where I ended up doing two people's jobs.'

'Before the late discovery, I used to think that this abuser was very skilled at finding ways to exploit my labour in such a way. I still hold this individual 100 per cent responsible for everything that happened but I now see that some of my autistic traits really made the ground extremely fertile for this abuse to take place.'

'I do not place any of the blame on myself, but I am now more cautious at work with supervisors or anyone else who may want to selfishly benefit from my work.'

'Friendships are a very complicated one for me. I struggle to understand friendship and where to draw the lines (close friend, friend, colleague, etc), what to share, how often to contact people or what to expect from them. I have spent considerable time talking with my therapist and reviewing my friendships since diagnosis.'

'I am a voracious reader and observe how friendships work in stories, how people around me interact and try hard not to overreach or overshare while being generous and supportive to the people I care about.'

'My mum sat me down to write a list of what I should look for in a relationship when I was 21 as I had a few disastrous ones and would be quite naïve and share contact details on train journeys and arrange to meet up. After my mum sat me down, I had some "rules", stuck to the list and met my neurodivergent husband.'

'Our strengths and challenges compliment each other, so it's a match made in heaven. Well, most of the time. I think some of my relationships on reflection prior to my mum's set of rules were probably verging on emotional abuse, there was often a lot of gaslighting within the relationship.'

There is a distinct lack of social and relational support and guidance for autistic women, yet we know that from hearing the experiences of women in our Late Discovered Community, coupled with the recent research that has been published, that autistic women and girls are at a significantly higher risk of sexual victimization when compared to the general population and are more likely to experience interpersonal victimization – from parents, friends, colleagues and loved ones.

And that has got to change.

And when you are repeatedly victimized, over a lifetime, it can mean living your life avoiding relationships, faces, spaces and places to keep yourself safe.

Not only that, you question your judgement.

You question your entire being and sense of self.

You can't work out why you are repeatedly harmed.

You carry with you trauma-related guilt and shame.

You feel guilty about disclosing to anyone what happened, a sense of betrayal towards an abuser for whom you promised to keep what happened to you a secret, out of fear.

And what guilt and shame does in this context is it wraps itself around you like cling film, a heavy, suffocating negative outer layer that tells you repeatedly that you're to blame, that you must be deserving of what has happened to you, shame silences you.

We know that guilt and shame in relation to trauma are also associated with a greater likelihood of experiencing suicidal ideation and suicide attempts in other populations (Tripp & McDevitt-Murphy, 2017). Could therefore our increased risk factor of suicide as late discovered autistic women in part be linked to our increased risk of abuse and interpersonal victimization, and if so, what are we doing on a societal level to minimize that risk? Who is studying it in relation to late discovered autistic women? Mental health, trauma and suicidality are themes we are going to explore a bit more in the next chapter.

I want to reassure you here that you are not to blame.

You are the victim.

The shame and guilt that has wrapped itself around you is not yours to carry.

I want you to know that I see you.

 EXPLORING *YOUR* SOCIAL AND RELATIONAL WORLD

There's a lot to unpack in this chapter and I hope that the stories and experiences shared by our Late Discovered Community will help you with exploring your own social and relational world.

Think about and reflect on your own communication style and preferences. If you really stopped to ask yourself what you need and what your preference is, what would that look like? What do you recognize about your friendships and relationships?

In your world, who are your safety anchors? Often by the time we have this late discovery we may have lost those people in our lives who assumed those roles for us growing up. The realization of that on top of grief and loss can hit us hard as we explore this brave new rediscovered world.

Conversely, it can hit home how we didn't have those safety anchors in our lives growing up and that too can lead to feelings of loss.

Bringing your attention to the here and now, who are the people you feel safe around? Who are your allies? What would be helpful to share with the people you love and care about when it comes to being more neuro-inclusive at home? How can they be more of an ally for you? What do you want them to know?

How has your late discovery impacted your social and relational world? What has changed? What have you learned about yourself?

And as you reflect on the experiences of abuse and interpersonal victimization you may feel a sense of heaviness, of experiences perhaps you've had but never spoken of, or felt a deep sense of shame about. If you are struggling with this chapter you can park it for now and come back to it when you feel ready to confront it. If you have someone in your life that you trust and can talk to who can hold that space (e.g. a therapist, close friend, family member), that could be an option for you to explore this together.

- What do you need to help you come home to yourself?

CHAPTER 10

Some of the Things We Don't Talk About Enough (But Need to Talk About More)

*Content warning: In this chapter I talk about suicide.

There are many things that we don't talk enough about, but need to talk about more (that could actually be a title for another book in itself) and there were multiple themes I wanted to explore in this chapter, but didn't have the word count to accommodate. That doesn't negate and dismiss the fact that they aren't important, but I would have been unable to do *all the themes* the justice they deserve in this chapter.

Even within the themes I have included here, I feel I've only scratched the surface. Some of the things we need to talk about more within the context of late discovery that I explore in this chapter are around our physical health, our mental health, trauma and suicidality, our sleep and the menopause.

Our physical health

Up until my late discovery I had never before connected together what appeared to be lots of individual chronic ill health issues which have blighted me since childhood, and no doctor had ever connected the dots, despite the (now) known prevalence between them and autism. In fact when I approached my GP for an autism assessment back in 2020, my 'long list' of ill health issues were never factored into the initial screening call as to whether I 'qualified' to be put on the autism assessment pathway – yet it seems obvious that our individual health stories should form part of the diagnostic assessment process.

A recent study led by a team of researchers at the University of Cambridge (Ward *et al.*, 2023) found that 'autistic people were more likely to have diagnosed medical conditions across all nine organ systems tested, compared to non-autistic people, and that autistic people had higher rates of 33 specific conditions compared to non-autistic peers' with several of the conditions including epilepsy and hypermobility, for example, relating to females only.

This is also the first epidemiological study to show that:

Ehlers-Danlos Syndrome (EDS) – a group of disorders that affects connective tissues and which cause symptoms such as joint hypermobility, loose joints that dislocate easily, joint pain and clicking joints, skin that bruises easily, extreme tiredness, digestive problems, dizziness, stretchy skin, wounds that are slow to heal, organ prolapse and hernias – may be more common among autistic women than non-autistic women.

'It was only when I was diagnosed and started reading voraciously about Autism that I came across Ehlers Danlos Syndrome, and again, everything in my past made sense. Joint pain, hypermobility, gut issues, skin healing and weight gain. It's frustrating in some ways as I was always looking for "cures", spending a fortune on treatment, physio, tests. Now I know that it's EDS (self-diagnosed as there's no specialists out here), and it's just part of me that I have to live with and find ways to manage it myself.'

The new research also replicates previous findings to show that autistic people have higher rates of all central sensitivity syndromes, which are a varied group of conditions that are related to dysregulation of the central nervous system, compared to non-autistic people. Central sensitivity syndromes include irritable bowel syndrome (IBS), temporomandibular joint syndrome (TMJ), migraine, tinnitus, myalgic encephalomyelitis/chronic fatigue syndrome (ME/CFS) and fibromyalgia.

'My whole life I've had stomach issues and I think this is massively due to the gut brain connection that we know about. I've also had regular bouts of depression and suicidal thoughts and I used to self-harm as a young adult. I've had a lot of CBT therapy and been on and off of antidepressants but they never work. I'm really sensitive to medication and none of them agreed with me.'

'I know now that it's quite common for Autistic people to be quite sensitive to medications and react to them. Whether it's because I'm so in tune with my body I can feel every slight pain or sensation and my mind runs away with me as to what it could be. It's quite debilitating at times as I hyperfocus on what I'm feeling.'

As part of my research for this book I interviewed my mum over several coffees to help fill in the gaps for me around the health issues I experienced as a small child that I had no recollection of. She explained that I developed epilepsy around the age of two years old, and one day found me passed out thinking that I was dead. It turned out that it was the childhood onset of epilepsy and what I was experiencing were epileptic seizures.

By the age of four I was prescribed anti-seizure medication which my body was sensitive to, and the doctors couldn't understand why 'because nobody else experienced these side effects'. I was later switched to Epilim which helped to control the seizures and they eventually stopped by the time I was eight years old.

We know now that compared with the general population, 'there is an increased prevalence of epilepsy in autistic people, and an increased prevalence of autism in epilepsy and that conditions such as ADHD, anxiety and sleep disorders are common in both epilepsy and autism' (Besag, 2018).

On top of that I had a speech delay as well as chronic ear infections and multiple operations to put grommets into my ears. I have vivid memories as a child of waking up with a burst eardrum and the contents on my pillow, and the excruciating pain it caused me – my mum can recall the level of pain it caused me too and how the pain would prevent me from sleeping and I would be constantly holding my ears, crying in pain, and as she advocated for me, she was labelled by health professionals in the 1980s a 'white coat mother' – an over-anxious mother exaggerating the pain her 'too sensitive' child was in.

It wasn't until recently that my mum requested a copy of her medical records that she found the term 'White Coat Syndrome' written in her medical notes – a label that a caring, advocating mother was given back in the 1980s that has stayed with her ever since. Perhaps this was the point at which I began to internalize my response to pain, and suppress the level of pain I was actually in. I can only imagine that as a child, in a room with multiple health professionals, being labelled 'too sensitive' and my mum 'over-anxious', the younger version of Catherine will have felt medically invalidated and gaslit, and protective of the harm being done to my mum.

The message I heard loud and clear from the medical world was that the pain I was experiencing wasn't valid, or real, or understood. There are parallels to my experience of chemotherapy, and how sensitive I was to the chemotherapy. I remember sitting down with my oncologist and drawing him a picture of all the parts of my body which were experiencing the brutal effects of the treatment.

From head to toe, my body was screaming at me, and despite explaining that I am autistic and that I'm highly sensitive to the effects of medication, nobody really got it. There were many dark times when I was anchored into the north face of the breast cancer mountain that I would have rather withdrawn myself from my treatment and taken the risk of survival without the trauma of chemo. I didn't feel listened to, seen or understood during this part of my treatment.

The only pull that kept me climbing the mountain and putting myself through the ordeal of 18 weeks of chemotherapy was my children. I had to be brave and continue on the route my oncologist had set out for me. I did, however, make the decision to stop after six cycles because my body had reached peak toxicity and couldn't tolerate any more of the treatment. What would have helped me during my treatment was a team (or a single health professional) who were autistic themselves or at the very least understanding of the intersecting layers of what it means to be autistic and having cancer, and unsurprisingly I couldn't find any research which explored the two.

Going back to being a child and the problems I had with my ears, as I was researching for this chapter I came across the Avon Longitudinal Study of Parents and Children (ALSPAC) which tracked the health of more than 14,000 children since birth and that of their parents from the early 1990s onwards. The study (Hall *et al.*, 2023) adds to the evidence that, 'compared with a typical population of the same age, early ear and upper respiratory symptoms are more common in those subsequently diagnosed with autism'.

My ear problems went hand in hand with repeated bouts of tonsillitis (my tonsils were later removed), as well as an egg allergy, along with various trips and falls as a child, which necessitated stitches in my chin and forehead, knocking out my front teeth, scalding myself, walking into a lamppost, a fractured collar bone and a nasty break in my wrist which had to be pinned back together again.

As a young adult I had many fainting episodes, the first happened at my very first gig due to being stood up for too long. I had to be pulled out by St Johns Ambulance. This was followed by several episodes on the train into work which would happen if I had to stand up, the most spectacular fainting episode was in my mid 20s at my daughter's assembly – that time I was whisked off to hospital in an ambulance. I never got to the bottom of *why* these episodes happened, rather I learned to not go to gigs, and to avoid standing up for long periods of time in any public place.

Young adulthood was the time that my gastro issues and UTIs (urinary tract infections) began too. I have suffered all my adult life with UTIs and subsequent kidney infections and have experienced agonizing pain that has seen me land in hospital with them and impacted my ability to show up for work – they have ruined all sorts of occasions. I was eventually referred to a urologist in my early 30s and diagnosed with urethral syndrome and was put on experimental drugs. I have also taken low dose antibiotics to try and prevent them, undergone urethral dilation surgery and done everything else I can to try and prevent them, but they still show up.

What I notice is that they show up in times of stress – my wedding day being one example. Whilst it was the happiest day of my life, it was also the most socially and sensory overloading day of my life. If I could go back in time with the knowledge I now have about myself I would have planned a very different wedding day.

I had my gallbladder removed in my early 20s after several episodes of acute cholecystitis and gallstones which necessitated hospital admissions, and ever since have suffered immensely with my stomach which my doctor put down to IBS (Irritable Bowel Syndrome). I have tried every 'diet' possible over the years to try and eliminate the debilitating symptoms I experience – from paleo to keto to eating very little – with little success. My gastro issues and chronic diarrhoea severely affects my quality of life and the availability of a toilet is never far from my mind.

Then there's my bendy body, which I now know to be hypermobility. By the time I hit my late 20s I had ripped the labrums from both my hip joints and was diagnosed with FAI (femoroacetabular impingement syndrome) which had resulted in the early onset of arthritis in my hips. My consultant spent my 30s trying to re-anchor the labrums back to my joints with multiple hip arthroscopies, and by the time I hit 40 my right hip had fractured and I underwent hip replacement surgery. Yet I am in more pain now than before my surgery with the added complication of now being left with a reduced femoral offset, leg length discrepancy, degenerative disc disease, several slipped discs and a curvature of my spine, and I know that my future holds more hip replacement surgery on both hips.

Some studies have suggested that hypermobility may increase the risk of developing FAI and labral tears, as the excessive motion of the hip joint can lead to instability and impingement. A recent study (Clapp *et al.*, 2021) found that 'hypermobility, or joint hyperlaxity, can result from inherited connective tissue disorders and these patients have a propensity to develop FAI syndrome and labral injury'.

Furthermore (Baeza-Velasco *et al.*, 2018) suggest that 'there is a growing body of research which suggests that both hypermobility and autism co-occur more often than expected than by chance'.

Months after my hip replacement surgery I developed chronic pain throughout my body which was diagnosed by my pain consultant as fibromyalgia – a chronic pain condition which limits me in so many ways along with MCAS (Mast cell activation syndrome), which is a 'malfunctioning' of part of the immune system. Then came my cancer diagnosis – my body has screamed enough, and chemotherapy has left me with debilitating peripheral neuropathy in my hands and feet on top of everything else, along with more medication to try and minimize the excruciating nerve pain I'm now in daily along with lymphoedema.

This is the first time I have confronted my 'long list' of health issues, and in writing about my health there is still a hesitation about saying how much pain I've been in for the last four decades – my default is to underplay everything, because I've been dismissed and disbelieved for so long. Now I can acknowledge and recognize that I've carried a lot of shame that isn't mine to keep carrying, and I can give myself permission now in this rediscovered world to let go of this.

This is my lived experience and my reality and that's ok. I class myself as disabled, just as many autistic people do in our community. It has taken me time to adjust to that and accept it.

I have a blue disabled badge yet so often feel shamed when I use it because of the invisibility of the aspects of my health. In one particular incident someone left a hurtful and derogatory note on my windscreen to tell me that I'm not disabled (despite my visible blue badge) and shouldn't take up the disabled parking space I was occupying – that devastated me at the time, pushing me into a very public overspill of tears and an aversion to ever using that car park or facility again. However, now I can see how ableist that act was.

Disability should not mean having to spend your life justifying accommodations to strangers, just because your disability doesn't match their preconceived notion of what disability *should* look like. My lived reality is that my whole body is in a constant daily state of pain, fatigue and discomfort, and my world has had to become smaller as a result – I need preparation and recovery time to 'participate' in things outside of my home, a well thought out plan that gets me from A to B in the least demanding way possible, and a variety of aids, support and accommodations to help me day to day.

I can't remember the last time I experienced a day without pain and fatigue. There are many things I used to be able to do that I took for granted that now feel out of reach because of the pain and extreme fatigue I will experience as a result, but I also don't want to *not* live and experience life, so I am committed to finding ways around so that I can, which has meant giving myself the permission to make and request whatever accommodations I need to enable that and to let go of the shame I've carried for this version of Catherine that I've become. Including supporting myself with a power chair for all the situations I find myself in where I need extra accommodations. Not because I've 'given up' or because I'm not 'trying hard enough' but so that my world doesn't have to remain so small, and so that I can regain some level of independence and live my life in less pain. I can honour my pain and choose to show up in a way that I am able.

One of the many challenges with invisible disabilities is that people don't see or understand what it's like to live with that level of pain and fatigue, and the energy that goes into navigating day-to-day life, and that even if you manage to do *the thing*, what people don't see is the scaffolding we have to put up to support doing *the thing* and the recovery we need post doing *the thing*.

There was a time when I would have to medicate to participate, however, medication is now a daily part of life. The 'exercise more' or 'push on through' and the 'you just need to try harder' messages are not the solutions everyone thinks when you live with chronic pain and fatigue – if only they were. This narrative is hugely ableist and deeply damaging because it's not about *trying harder.*

Exercise was such an integral part of my life, I used to live to run, and throughout my 20s I ran and raced in some beautiful places, which I now have stashed in my memory bank. The loss I feel from no longer being able to do the activities that once brought me so much joy fills me with sadness, but thankfully I have found alternative ways to 'move' my body.

My body is finally being listened to.

It had to scream at me to hear it, and dragged me up a breast cancer mountain when there was nothing in the tank.

And had I known about the co-occurrence of all of these conditions and autism, maybe it would have given me a narrative and understanding whereby I could have minimized some of my health struggles, or at the very least I could have not tried to plough on through my life thinking that those struggles were just part and parcel of life, and berating myself for finding things so difficult.

Maybe I could have been kinder to myself and more compassionate.

Maybe I would have been listened to by my doctors, my pain seen and validated, rather than experiencing the shame I've felt for having so much going on, and instead putting up and shutting up.

But what matters is that I'm listening now; I'm tuned in and I've connected the dots, and rather than constantly pushing my body to its limits, I'm giving it the kindness and level of nurturing that it needs and deserves through the adaptations I make for myself, the accommodations I now seek out and the slower pace I'm taking in this rediscovered world. This is courageous compassion in action.

It's ok to say out loud that I struggle with chronic pain and fatigue, and that I need aids and support – neither of those things mean that I am less than.

And neither of those things mean that you are less than.

You are worthy and deserving of love.

I am worthy and deserving of love.

Even on the days when it's hardest, we are worthy and deserving of love.

You are deserving of love that meets you where you are at, and grows with you as you are becoming. Love that is all encompassing of the beautiful human that you are.

Take this as a gentle reminder to not forget who you are and what you are deserving of.

Mental health, trauma and suicidality

Autism is not a mental health condition, nor is it a mental illness, yet people often think it is, and treat it as if it is. We do, however, know that autistic people are *more likely* to experience symptoms of mental ill health and to be diagnosed with a mental health condition.

'I have had difficulties with my mental health for as long as I remember. I have complex PTSD due to attachment and relational trauma and emotional bullying.'

When we look at co-occurrence, it's estimated that between 12 and 30 per cent of autistic people have a co-occurring learning disability and approximately a third report a diagnosed mental health condition. Additionally, other neurodevelopmental conditions often co-occur with autism, for example, ADHD has been found to have a lifetime prevalence of 40.2 per cent in autistic people (NHS England, 2023). Anecdotally, Autism and ADHD (AuDHD) appears to be a common co-occurrence in our late discovered community, with either one being the first diagnosis followed swiftly by the other.

Mental ill health is a significant aspect of increased mortality for autistic adults, with autistic adults up to nine times more likely than non-autistic adults to experience suicidal ideation (NHS England, 2023).

Furthermore, a recent meta-analysis (Steenfeldt-Kristensen *et al.*, 2020) shows that self-injurious behaviour is more common in autistic people, 'with a prevalence rate of 42%, which is significantly higher than prevalence estimates for the general population (5.9%)'. This means that the prevalence of self-injurious behaviour is 42 per cent higher among autistic people than among non-autistic people. The authors of the meta-analysis make reference to the fact that in order to explore the association between gender and self-injury further, that future research needs to include more female autistic participants.

A recent study undertaken by a team of researchers in the UK found that high autistic traits are found in adults who have attempted suicide (Cassidy *et al.*, 2022). This is the first study to explore potentially undiagnosed autism and attempt to quantify autistic traits through coroners' records in those who have died by suicide.

We know that autistic adults are up to seven times more likely to die by suicide than non-autistic adults and that the relative risk may be greater for autistic people with co-occurring ADHD and for late diagnosed/discovered autistic women, who have been found to be 13 times more likely than non-autistic women to die by suicide (NHS England, 2023).

However, there is also recognition that further research is needed to ensure a greater understanding of potential gender differences to include transgender and nonbinary autistic people, with a call for clarity to advance suicide prevention for the whole autistic community (Kirby *et al.*, 2024).

If we feel and experience the world too much, it makes sense that we will experience trauma and traumatic events more intensely too. Add in a lifetime of being marginalized, stigmatized, misunderstood and never feeling like we belong, then that trauma becomes cumulative. Through my work, I see an almost universally experienced correlation of trauma in late discovered autistic women – our trauma is so often multilayered and multi-faceted. The most shocking discovery is that I have yet to meet an autistic woman who hasn't experienced repeated traumas throughout their life

In two recent studies on trauma and autism, the first one (Haruvi-Lamdan *et al.*, 2020) showed that autistic people show an increased risk of experiencing potentially traumatic events. The second study (Happé *et al.*, 2020) shows us that the *type* of trauma that autistic people experience often doesn't look like the trauma that we see described in the DSM-5, which means that people on the outside don't often see or understand the trauma that autistic people encounter in their day-to-day lives. Our experiences are invalidated, dismissed and invisible to others – the antithesis of a trauma-informed approach.

Furthermore, many of the life events experienced as traumas would not be recognized in some current diagnostic systems, raising concerns that autistic people may not receive the help they need for likely PTSD.

Add in the way our minds are able to hyperfocus, and our ability for pattern spotting and need for sense making, our need for safety and to feel understood, as well as sensory and emotional processing related to the traumatic event, you can start to understand why we're more at risk of experiencing many life events and day-to-day interactions as traumatic and why those traumatic events are all consuming and overwhelming, and why we might find avoidance, shutdown and repression the coping mechanisms we lean into, and why burnout is so prevalent – our bodies eventually scream enough to us, and those traumas (issues) become stored in our tissues – and why we have higher prevalence rates of mental health and suicide amongst the autistic population

However, what neither of these studies explore are the specific trauma experiences through the lens of autistic women, or those from marginalized genders.

Why are health professionals not making the connection between poor mental health, suicidality and the prevalence of decades of trauma in late discovered autistic women and people?

Why is nobody outraged by the extent of trauma experiences

of autistic women and people to make researching it (and funding that research) a priority?

Why are our experiences not being heard or understood?

Faces, spaces and places

Trauma imprints itself on our bodies and our minds, and in response we measure all future events in relation to the trauma. Will this face, space or place keep me safe or take me back to a place of danger? As safety seekers it makes sense that the more we experience trauma, and the cumulative effects of trauma over the lifespan, the more we avoid, mask, shutdown and in my case, *flight* my way to safety.

It might be a workplace that has caused us harm, an experience we've had in a particular place or space, or an individual who has unleashed that harm. Whatever it is, our association with that face, space or place then becomes something we don't ever want to feel or be reminded of ever again.

What we see and what we experience is that social, relational and sensory trauma is so often dismissed by others, we're labelled 'drama queens' for making a 'big' thing of it, or we hear that we just need to 'get over it' (the double empathy problem in action) yet no amount of 'forced' exposure lessens the pain.

To find safety in our worlds, to cope and survive, we make our worlds smaller and smaller as a protective measure, and in the process isolate ourselves, which in turn further compounds poor mental health and wellbeing, or conversely as we heard in Chapter 8, we may have no option but to heavily mask as a safety response, putting ourselves in the path of harm. That's a heavy survival strategy to have to attempt to maintain – and for whom?

Who does that serve?

Sleep

Sleep has always been a challenge for me, but it's also something I've sought to fiercely protect my need for since my late discovery. My brain often comes alive and is at its most creative at night. It resists bedtime with a vengeance, and instead wants to take me on a deep dive expedition – this book had mostly been written between the hours of 8pm and 12pm. I have to be mentally exhausted, my neurons no longer firing, I imagine that they have to become like smouldering embers on a fire before I can fall asleep, and no amount of camomile tea or warm baths can dial down my active brain.

Some of my earliest memories are of having night terrors, of sitting bolt upright in bed and screaming, and those haunting night terrors and vivid dreams where I feel like I've lived a lifetime all in one sleep cycle have continued into my adult sleep world, although interestingly since my rediscovery I've not had a single night terror, the vivid, lived a lifetime in one sleep cycle dreams, however, have persisted.

Being scared of the dark, a hypersensitivity to noise, the wrong sort of light, temperature, smell, the feel of the bedding, and clutter are the things that disrupt my sleep, as are the different and conflicting circadian rhythms in my neurodivergent family. If I'm sleeping somewhere that isn't home, the environment is never 'just right'.

If I don't get enough sleep, it affects my speech, working memory and pretty much my whole sense of functioning, and my pain levels. I average about six hours of sleep per night, but know that my body craves more. The struggle I have is in getting my brain to power down, and I'm not sure that it ever does, it has an overabundance of energy and I have to be absolutely exhausted to daytime nap.

As part of my chemotherapy treatment I was prescribed steroids which made me feel wired, resulting in an even more active brain and insomnia at a time when my body needed sleep more than ever to heal, repair and regenerate those healthy cells. This was never addressed or understood by my oncology team.

In a study (Pavlopoulou & Dimitriou, 2018), over 70 per cent of autistic adults said they experienced difficulty falling asleep or staying asleep, associating this with sensory issues and high anxiety, and around half were unable to stay asleep for long, whilst four in ten experienced nightmares.

'I struggle staying asleep: anything and everything can wake me up (lights, sounds, smells, etc). I also can't sleep during the day even when I have the time to do it. I have always had extremely vivid and complex dreams; my friends and relatives have always made fun of the "weird and crazy" dreams that I have. Rarely a day goes by when I don't have intense dreams. They aren't necessarily nightmares or scary or sad, but they are super complex with many twists and turns and a lot of characters and situations.'

Despite sleep being such a central component of our frequency circle, it's not something that really registered for me until my rediscovery. I have since experimented with different sleep aids (eye mask, earphones, black out blinds, sleep meditations, calm uncluttered space etc) to help reduce sensory sensitivity and I have concluded that my circadian rhythm doesn't fit with the way the world is set up to function.

I'm not an early bird; I'm a night owl, and the compassionate conclusion is to design my life more around my natural rhythm with sleep tuned into *my* frequency, not the normative imposed rhythm imposed on me, working with my natural rhythm, rather than against it. The challenge, however, is that society isn't designed around the night owls and there are expectations and demands that we live our lives swimming against the tide of what we actually need.

But in acknowledging and understanding our sleep patterns, natural circadian rhythms and needs, we are empowered to do more of what we need, to make those adaptations, and to seek out the accommodations we need to get a good night's sleep, and ultimately optimize our frequency by working with ourselves, rather than against ourselves. Because sleep matters a lot when it comes to our mental and physical health and wellbeing, and it's something that the world of chronobiology is exploring more and more.

How do we then honour our needs of our natural circadian rhythm so that it works for us, rather than against us?

How *can you* honour your needs even when they conflict with others?

Menopause – When the wheels start to fall off

There is very little out there when it comes to autism and the menopause and how we navigate the menopausal transition, or in my case, crash into menopause at 43 years old as a side effect of my cancer – there was no 'transition' rather the onset of symptoms happened overnight. Yet we know from the lived experiences within our Late Discovered Community that at every hormonal crunch point from menstruation, pregnancy, post-natal, perimenopause, menopause and post-menopause, we struggle.

> 'My late discovery came about because of a perfect storm. As cited in the scientific article by Rachel Moseley, my autism "broke" during menopause. A number of life events collided in a short space of time and I unravelled. I had physical and psychological health issues and ran out of energy to mask. My husband asked for a divorce. I told him if I was him I would divorce me, I knew I was unbearable. I didn't want to be me. I considered self-harm, running away and suicide.'

It makes sense that if we experience the world differently that we are going to feel the effects of fluctuating hormones differently too – everything from our emotional regulation, sleep, mental health and our individual sensory sensitivities.

And whilst there was generic information available during my cancer treatment around menopause, and workshops on offer, there wasn't anything specific about the autistic experience of cancer-induced menopause. There was nothing available about the autistic experience of cancer full stop. The autistic perspective when it comes to menopause (peri and post inclusive) is generally missing from the mainstream; the autistic going through cancer *and* menopause is missing entirely, with the added complication of not being able to take HRT due to the effects of cancer. I'm not the first autistic woman to go through both cancer and menopause hand in hand, and I won't be the last.

I've already talked in this chapter and previous chapters about how as autistic women we are more vulnerable to suicide, chronic ill health and mental health, and we've explored in previous chapters how we experience the world, our emotions and our cognitive worlds – when you layer all this up and add in menopause it's no wonder we hear it described in our community as the point in our lives when 'the wheels to start to fall off', and why for many women, menopause is the point of their autistic self-discovery.

Not one single study existed on the menopause in autism until 2020, when an online discussion (focus group) with seven autistic women was undertaken (Moseley *et al.*, 2020). The study found that:

> Autism-related difficulties (including sensory sensitivity, socialising with others and communicating needs) were reported to worsen during the menopause, often so dramatically that some participants suggested they found it impossible to continue to mask their struggles. Participants also reported having extreme meltdowns, experiencing anxiety and depression, and feeling suicidal highlighting how important it is that professionals pay attention to menopause in autism, and discusses future research directions.

Listening to our community, we need autism-specific menopause support and interventions, and for our specific challenges and our vulnerabilities during menopause to suicide and mental health to be understood by health professionals, our families, our communities and within the workplace.

We need to do so much more.

 EXPLORING *YOUR* EXPERIENCES

- As you've read through this chapter, what has resonated for you? What struggles have you had with your physical health throughout your life? Have you ever associated 'what' you feel in your body with being autistic?

- And what would help you to be more compassionately aware?

- What message would you like to share with those around you about the things you struggle with? What support do you need from yourself and from others?

- When you look back on your mental health and your current mental health what are some of the things you struggle with?

If you've not already explored past trauma and PTSD, now might be the time, if you feel ready, to search out someone who could guide you through that. Look for someone who is trauma-informed and neuro-inclusive in their approach. Or explore the ways to process your experiences which you find helpful.

- Thinking about your sleep, do you get enough quality sleep?

- What are your sleep challenges and what interferes with your sleep?

- What happens when you don't get enough sleep and what helps when you are sleep deprived?

- Do you have a sleep pattern?

- And finally if you are perimenopausal or post-menopausal, can you recognize how it is/has impacted you? What do you need from others around you (i.e. loved ones, work, health professionals) and how can you extend more compassionate awareness to yourself?

CHAPTER 11

Workplaces We Thrive in

In this chapter we explore the challenges we face in the workplace as autistic women, the things that help us thrive, along with what more needs to be done to create neuro-inclusive workplaces. We explore struggle clashes, safety anchors and strength nurturing and what that looks like and feels like for you.

We also hear from leading employment lawyer and Season One podcast guest, Ed Jenneson, who shares his expertise and experience with you in the form of a Q&A to help empower you and arm you with the legal knowledge that we should all have access to, and Kirsty Cullen-Campanelli, a Season Two podcast guest on the 'how to' create autistic inclusive workplaces.

As autistic women, we have so many skills to offer, yet face a mountain of challenges in the workplace. The UK Office for National Statistics (2021) reported that only 22 per cent of autistic people were in work, the lowest among the disabilities they analysed, which means that autistic people still face the highest rates of unemployment of all disabled groups.

Off the back of these statistics, the charity Autistica here in the UK has committed to undertaking research in collaboration with University College London (UCL), to find solutions so that by 2030 more autistic people can thrive in the workplace. Some of the women in our community are forced out of the workplace and into self-employment, freelance and/or contract roles because they are misunderstood and unsupported in the workplace. Bullying, abuse and interpersonal victimization is also a common experience, and the weight of cumulative trauma is often the tipping point, with others crashing out of the workforce altogether.

Many of our community members find themselves in a state of burnout and can no longer work; many are struggling with chronic ill health and mental health challenges, are homeschooling neurodivergent children, or cannot find work they can do from home that fits around school hours/caring responsibilities, or they are supporting their children who can't *not won't* go to school some days, or who can't access before and after school provision due to support needs.

Actively seeking autistic women

In 2022, the British intelligence agency GCHQ and weapons manufacturer BAE Systems issued appeals to attract more neurodivergent women to work for them in cybersecurity jobs, actively seeking autistic women to address gaps in their workforces. Why aren't we seeing other employers, across other sectors falling over themselves to actively attract, recruit and retain autistic women employees?

Attracting autistic women to fill a skills gap is one thing, but any programme or organization that is looking to attract autistic talent, or who employs autistic people, really needs to build in the foundations from the outset when it comes to retention, belonging, inclusion and burnout prevention.

It starts with recruitment – it's in the way you interview, and how the process is designed, the language you use, the ways you work, the safety you create, the support you give, and the accommodations you are *willing* to make, and saying what those are.

It's not about having a blanket 'neurodiversity' policy which simply pays lip service to being inclusive by naming a long list of marginalized neurodivergent groups without actually saying how it will meet people's individual needs.

Within your policy, commit to creating, understanding and supporting communities of interest – across all areas of your business from floor to board – and not just during awareness days/weeks.

Getting someone in to talk about autism once a year isn't being neuro-inclusive.

Be committed to being micro-focused and make it your mission to understand the very real intersectional challenges facing autistic women and people in the workplace, and make your workplace the kind of safe and supportive space where your autistic employees are able to disclose without fear and are able to thrive to their full potential.

A community of interest might, for example, be *late discovered autistic women.*

- Do you have safe spaces for them to connect?

- Do you understand the challenges they face in the workplace? What are some of the key themes?

- Do you understand the intersectional challenges they face in the workplace?

- Do you understand what support mechanisms might help in the workplace?

- Do you regularly listen to their experiences and learn from their experiences?

- How can you better support them right across the lifespan? How might support need to be flexible and adapatable?

- How can you take a person-centred approach based on individual need?

- Do you have safe places and faces in your organization? What might that look like?

- Are your HR teams and managers trauma informed?

Another community of interest might be *parents of neurodivergent children.*

- Do you have safe spaces for parents of neurodivergent children to connect?

- Do you know how many people in your organization are parents to neurodivergent children?

- Do you understand what the challenges are for parents of neurodivergent children?

- How can you better support them?

- How can you listen to their experiences and better tailor support?

This approach doesn't just signal psychological and emotional safety, it shows you care about neuro-inclusion, about your people. It shows that you are an ally. That you want to do better. That you want to continuously learn from experience. It makes you stand out in a sea of workplaces that just don't get it.

'My extreme attention to detail and the way in which I can categorize information and do analysis is definitely my biggest autistic strength. This helps me be an extremely organized planner in my personal life in situations such as travel but also it helps me thrive conducting research and doing overall knowledge management which is what I do for a living. Added to that – the fact that I have managed to work in a sphere that is deeply connected to one of my biggest special interests has given me a "superpower" at work.'

Safety seeking

My work is now so niched and outed in the autistic experience that there is (virtually) no safety requirement to have to hide behind a mask anymore, and I've worked hard to make those shifts and changes. The vast majority of the work that I do is now delivered from my home, on a screen via Zoom, which means that my working environment is fully accommodating of my needs, but it also means I'm isolated and spend the majority of my day with just me, myself and I.

For the last 18 months I've been delivering training remotely on the NHS National Autism Trainer Programme, hired because I am autistic, and a space where I'm training NHS mental health professionals in their inpatient and community mental health setting on how to deliver more person centred, neuro-affirming care for their autistic patients. I'm hired to show up as my whole autistic self, and I cannot tell you how liberating it is to be able to show up to work as me – to be able to bring my whole self to my work.

I'm able to request accommodations from my co-facilitator and for my needs to be accommodated. To openly stim with my fidget toy as I'm presenting to help soothe my nervous system and that being ok, and to talk openly with mental health professionals about my inside world as an autistic woman, and to have the autonomy to create the environment I can thrive in.

When Covid hit, the world had to pivot and change, which means remote work is now more mainstream and far more acceptable. I look back now on my career and wonder how I ever coped with a daily commute, the travel, an open plan office and the pressure of eye contact and the reliance on working memory (which always failed to show up for me) when presenting in person.

I remember my first graduate job in Local Government after finishing university and being asked to present some findings from a survey to a room full of important people and not being able to remember what I was there to talk about. I remember the humiliation and embarrassment I felt as I stood there silent, unable to talk, everybody looking at me, until my flight response kicked in and I ran out the room, mortified by the fact that I couldn't do what others were doing.

Part of climbing the ladder in my career (which I did but at a cost to my health) was to be able to present in meetings with little to no preparation and excel in interviews without any script or notes. I always felt that whilst I stood out on paper, I was a let-down when it came to performing, especially at interviews – my memory recall failed me time and time again.

Yet writing strategies, connecting and building solid relationships with partners, influencing people and policy, being able to translate the big picture into something tangible and understandable, big idea generation and finding creative solutions to complex problems were where my strengths sat. I can now look back at these experiences through my autistic affirming lens and extend some compassion and understanding to myself.

I didn't fail in these situations, rather the *situations failed me* – they failed to take into account my cognitive processing and the way that my neurotype works, and that with support and accommodations, I know now that I *can* excel at interviews, and speak in person with great clarity and authority to audiences of over 7000 people and that what I say connects with those audiences.

I know because I have that now in my self-employed evidence bank. Coming home to myself has meant now knowing *what* supports I need, *how* I need to work, and crucially *why* – unleashing my potential and no longer being held back by limitations placed upon me.

It's been making work work for me, in the way that I need.

And I wonder what making work work for you looks like?

What do you need?

Struggle clashing

Pre-discovery I wasn't strength nurturing, I was struggle clashing, and that is an exhausting way to operate. It's like asking me to show up at work every day and write with my left hand, when I'm actually right-handed. My inner narrative with left hand writing is always going to be 'must try harder' and 'why is this so hard for me?' And no matter how many times I attempt to write left-handed it *always* feels hard.

I don't want my life to be about struggle clashing and for it to feel harder than it needs to be. In that chapter of my life I heavily masked and compensated to get me through the daily onslaught of showing up to work to do my job, and wherever possible I used scripts to get me through. It was eventually my body screaming 'enough' that ultimately saw me exit full-time paid employment in my early 30s from a career as a health strategist that I'd put my all into.

Out of necessity I had to find a way of strength nurturing and, for me, the only way of creating such an environment was to work for myself.

> 'I left my planned career in teaching for a lot of reasons, many of which were related to being autistic. I found the classroom to be a very overstimulating environment at times, as well as struggling to reconcile my personal views with the rules and examination processes I was required to perpetuate. The overwork and lack of free weekends led to constant burnout too.'

Safety anchors

I have several *safety anchors* in my work; these are adaptations and accommodations I have made to support my struggles, and these are non-negotiable. These are my burnout prevention strategies at work.

Co-facilitating and co-delivering

Delivering training or a workshop with a *chosen* co-trainer or co-facilitator. Knowing that there is a safe person there to support me whilst I'm doing my thing makes it possible to do.

Scripts

If I'm delivering a presentation or speaking on a podcast I want to have my script/notes in front of me. Just as someone needs their glasses when they cannot see, I need the words I want to say.

In advance interviews and meetings

I only do interviews where I receive the questions in advance, where I can think about what I want to say, and have the script in front of me. Interviews, exams and meetings shouldn't be a test of my memory recall ability but rather the opportunity for me to show what I know and what I can bring.

My workspace

I need complete quiet to work, without distraction, and a space that is visually sensory soothing. And if I'm working in a different environment, I need my support requests to be accommodated and factored in. If 'in person' delivery is needed, I need planning and decompression time, and a carefully planned travel itinerary that takes into account and accommodates both my physical and multiply neurodivergent needs.

Preparation, recovery and reflection time

Whatever I'm doing I need time to prepare, recover and reflect and I ensure that this is factored into my day and week.

Time blocking

I need to know what I'm doing, when I'm doing it and for how long – this helps me to prepare, and I struggle with too many different systems, apps, or overly complicated platforms which are supposed to help you. An extension of the 'too many steps' involved in something and my brain hits a wall.

Autonomy over the how, what and when

Having 'set' days for the different elements of my work matters too. I need routine and predictability and the conditions and environment where I can deep dive. Having autonomy and full control over my diary matters, and if there are too many demands on my time I very quickly become overwhelmed. I need time to recover and decompress, along with whole blocks of time in my dairy where there are no demands on me. I've learned the hard way what my 'safe' limits are to prevent burnout.

'Autonomy is crucial for me. I have a strong need to tackle projects in my own way and I get hugely frustrated when others try to micro-manage me. I've gone freelance so that I can be my own boss.'

Strength nurturing

And I am *strength nurturing* by focusing on my strengths in my work, and enveloping myself in the work I'm most passionate about.

Hosting a podcast is my happy place. Creating that safe space for my guests and holding that space for stories to be told is deep diving for me. And the very nature of podcasting means that I can utilize all my safety anchors *and* strength nurture and manage to reach listeners in over 120 countries worldwide.

I spent three years as the resident therapist on BBC Local Radio and it meant I got to go on air and talk to thousands of listeners, but without the pressure of doing it script less. Just me and the presenter in the studio having a conversation with each other, which just so happened to be live and on air.

Delivering training and workshops, hosting panel discussions, facilitating The Late Discovered Club Group Circles and writing books (I say 'books' because this might be the first but it definitely isn't the last) is playing to my strengths and supporting my struggles in equal measures.

However, what people don't see is the amount of planning, preparation, scripting, decompressing, recovery and constant burnout prevention strategies that go on behind the scenes to enable me to show up and do what I do, and the isolation I experience in response to the solitary working environment and life I've had to create and design for myself so that I can show up and do the work that I want to do and that I'm passionate about, to support and be present for my children in the way they need *and* make a living.

As I look back on my career over the last 25 years, I can see that I have made some courageous decisions and bold moves to create a workplace that I can thrive in. Some of those decisions I made intuitively, and reactively in the midst of burnout, but now that I know what my struggle clashes are, and the safety anchors I need, my career decisions are very deliberate.

And my new mantra?

If the juice isn't worth the squeeze, say no, and say it loudly.

'From a neurodivergent perspective I think I've been really lucky – I chose a career that worked really well for me. It plays to my passions and superpowers, and I've always been a super high performer because I enjoyed it and was good at it. I would say that being a working mum was more of a hindrance than my neurodivergence.'

'That said, at the end of my corporate career I was completely undone by office politics. I found it abhorrent and went against my deep instilled sense of justice. It was a big deciding factor in leaving – I felt like I was being asked to support the agendas of the few rather than do the right things that would make the most impact. I couldn't rationalize that, I stopped enjoying what I was doing, and then I couldn't be as good at my job. And If I couldn't enjoy it or have the impact then frankly, I didn't want to do it.

So, I left, and now while I find self-employment a massive change and challenge, I really enjoy being able to direct my energy at clients where I think I can have the most fun and the biggest impact.'

Knowledge is power

In Season One of the podcast I was joined by Ed Jenneson, an expert employment law solicitor and a leading voice in the neurodiversity space as a result of his diagnosis of ADHD and dyslexia as an adult. Ed came on the podcast to share his journey of discovery and to contribute his insights in relation to the Equality Act 2010 and how it *should* work in practice.

We asked our Late Discovered Community for three of their burning questions for Ed to address in this book to help empower you, and arm you with the legal knowledge that you should have access to.

What is classed as a reasonable adjustment at work?

The employee should share (i) what they are struggling with and (ii) how the employer can help to reduce the struggle. That is (in a nutshell) a request for an adjustment. The employer will then determine if it is reasonable.

Sometimes an employee will not know what they need the employer to do to help them reduce the disadvantages. This can be navigated together, using Occupational Health or other treating physicians. Having said that, the employee should always know what they are struggling with and that should be the focus. If an employee can articulate that, a conversation about how the employer can help should follow.

An employee can advocate their struggles relating to almost anything in the workplace and that is likely to amount to a request for an adjustment. Obvious things such as contract terms, including start times, finish times and rest breaks. It can also include policies and procedures that may require adjusting – such as attendance in the office or performance targets.

What is more difficult for the parties to articulate is the informal policies or arrangements which require adjusting – those not written down anywhere. For example, (all taken from real cases) the requirement for hot desking; open plan working; travel; the use of headphones; working from home; texting instructions; the requirement to work in teams; the requirement for all staff to attend social events and/or a requirement for reading text in a particular font or format (and many many others not even thought of yet!).

After an employee and employer have determined what the employee is finding difficult, the next thing is they must consider what would reduce the disadvantage (the struggle) for the employee and whether that reduction is reasonable. An employee must show that it would make it better for them in a way which is not 'trivial'.

Provided an employee is clear that the requested adjustment will reduce the disadvantage (e.g. if you speak the instructions rather than text them I will understand them), the employer must make the adjustment unless it is unreasonable to do so. Whether it is reasonable will be determined by the burden the adjustment places upon the employer. Examples given where an employer can refuse are:

- it is too expensive

- it doesn't really work, i.e. it does not really reduce the disadvantage

- it is too difficult or inefficient

- it doesn't fit in with the nature or culture of the business

- size of the business, i.e. there are insufficient resources.

As many adjustments are relatively minor, provided the employee has demonstrated it should reduce the difficulty they face, the adjustment should often be made or trialled.

Do I need to have a formal autism diagnosis to request adjustments?

No. It will be easier to say that the employer has the required knowledge if there is a formal diagnosis but if an employee is presenting themselves as autistic an employer should involve Occupational Health (there are specialist neurodivergent organizations who can assist).

An employee is 'disabled' (the term used in the Equality Act 2010) from the date that they became disabled, rather than the date of a formal diagnosis. It could therefore be the case that an employee does not have a formal diagnosis until they begin tribunal proceedings – or it could be nothing more than an opinion rather than a diagnosis.

Ultimately it is for a tribunal to decide on the question of 'disability'. If an employee does not have a formal diagnosis, they should focus their efforts on articulating the impact on their normal day-to-day activities. They should explain to the employer what they find difficult throughout the day (not limited simply to work). This is what a tribunal will consider when determining the issue in the future. An employee should explain that the difficulties faced are not 'minor' or 'trivial'.

If an employee presents this information, an employer would

not be wise to say 'we don't believe you' without taking reasonable steps to ascertain the position. In fact, the Equality Code states that 'an employer must do all they reasonably can to find out if the worker has a disability' and that an employer should have appropriate systems in place for disclosure and to maintain an employee's dignity and confidentiality at all times.

Do I need to legally self-disclose that I am autistic?

There is no specific legal obligation for you to disclose and you cannot get into trouble for not disclosing (although it will be more difficult to allege a failure if you don't at least indicate to your employer you are autistic). You also cannot get into trouble for disclosing late. For example, if you decide to disclose during employment rather than at the start, an employer cannot take a negative view for a late disclosure.

There should be no 'cons' but I live in the real world so of course there are some. You may be met with a lack of understanding from other people and even negative reactions. You may even suffer prejudice, bullying, failure to make adjustments, heavy handed sanctions or denied promotion.

In terms of protection, an employee is protected by the Equality Act 2010. This includes protection from harassment, direct and indirect discrimination and a requirement for the employer to make reasonable adjustments. You don't need to wait until after employment has terminated before you claim – or you don't even need to be offered a job or even an interview before a claim can be issued.

Autistic-affirming and inclusive workplaces

One of the many challenges that our late discovered autistic community faces is the need for more autistic-affirming and inclusive workplaces that feel like safe places in which to self-disclose and create the safety anchors we need individually to prevent overwhelm, burnout and ill health.

This has featured in almost every single story I've explored on the podcast, because without psychologically safe workplaces, we mask, and masking leads to burnout, and burnout affects our mental and physical health and wellbeing and we end up excluded and exiting workplaces because they *can't and won't* accommodate our individual needs.

There are a number of ways late discovered autistic women are discriminated against in the workplace:

- We know that many women are unable to access a formal diagnosis because of the many barriers we explored in Chapter 2 and that many workplaces exclude support and accommodations without a formal diagnosis.

- There is a mass misunderstanding of what autism is, and how it presents from floor to board level. Organizations think that a catch all 'neurodiversity policy' or celebrating an awareness day is doing enough. The reality is we need to educate specifically about what autism is and what it isn't, deconstruct the stereotypes, de-stigmatize language and centre the experiences of autistic women in the workplace. It's often this lack of knowledge and understanding that creates conflicts in the workplace – the double empathy problem in practice.

- When accommodations are requested they are often seen as being 'awkward' and 'too demanding' and the knock-on effect is that relationships change, bullying begins, career progression becomes stifled and that thwarted sense of belonging deepens. Burnout, poor mental and physical health is often the outcome and we see a mass exodus of autistic potential from the workplace.

- An intersectional identity can and does create barriers that autistic people face in the workplace, e.g. being an autistic woman who is also gender non-conforming, who might also be a woman of colour, who might also be disabled. There are many late discovered autistic women in our community who talk about their experiences of being multiply disadvantaged because of their intersectional identity.

So what should employers be doing to overcome this?

According to Ed:

> employers should focus on creating safety for *all* its workforce. An environment where its workers are not afraid to be who they are and say how they feel. The ability for employees to say what they require to have their needs met.
>
> An environment that results in not living with worry, including fear of their attachment to colleagues being damaged or destroyed if they disclose and that they do not fear their job prospects (or even their roles) will be at risk if they share. That sounds simplistic and something all employers should already be doing – but it is not as there is such a huge array of needs across the workforce.

Ed shares his top tips *for employers* as a starting point:

- Invite actually autistic women and people to talk to staff, and not just as part of an awareness day.

- Communicate and reassure employees that there will be no negative consequences if they do disclose.

- Employers should take note about the use of language, and why educating all staff on the neurodiversity paradigm is essential.

- The businesses that are incredibly profitable should be driving best practices. That is why working collaboratively with employers is so important. We can achieve so much more together rather than as individuals.

Kirsty Cullen-Campanelli, a Season Two podcast guest further adds that to create autistic inclusive workplaces, 'we need to get to *know* our workforce, our people'. She says:

> It's important that in order to support our late discovered autistic women in the workplace – we are open and lead with empathy. This includes being open to accommodations. Focusing on the can, not the can't, and promoting kindness.

To get granular for a moment, this could look like:

- Deconstructing stereotypes through education on autistic women, by autistic women

- Prioritizing leading with empathy as a core pillar

- Mentoring and advocacy programs for support

- Include autistic people in the discussion of how their strengths can be brought to a role

- Consider simple changes to work environment (i.e. dimmer switches for lights, offering quiet/sensory rooms, designated workspace)

- Design more sensory supportive workplaces – involve autistic people in the design

- Building protocols around workflows and environments that are inclusive, such as:

  o Ensuring clear directives are a baseline, to follow up with written clarity of those directives

  o Allowing time to digest and decompress between meetings

  o Ensuring agendas are shared ahead of time

  o Considering hybrid working or working from home.

Kirsty says that 'Creating psychological safety leads to higher performance and greater job satisfaction – that's a fact.'

But what does it mean?

Kirsty explains that:

at its core, psychological safety is about creating an environment where people can speak up, share ideas, ask questions, share feedback – and make mistakes without fear. Whether that fear be of humiliation, marginalised, embarrassed or retribution. Creating a psychologically safe environment supports *genuine* participation and contribution by people as they will feel valued and respected.

So, how do we create such an environment?

Kirsty believes that:

> it starts with talking about it. With conversations, with information, with education. To create inclusive workspaces, we have to start with removing the stigma, and 'otherness'. And that work needs to be done by the workplaces that we're part of.

Kirsty shares that:

> It has been one of the most terrifying experiences of my life disclosing on such a mass scale – because there is stigma. There is stigma about talking about oneself, there is stigma in being less than, there is stigma in being broken, there is stigma in being disabled, and non-neurotypical, because that's the way society is set up. But it's changing, and we are part of that, and autistic inclusion is everyone's responsibility.

 ## WORKPLACES THAT *YOU* THRIVE IN

I hope that this chapter will have given you some food for thought about what it means to thrive as an autistic person in the workplace. Thinking about your own experience, what are/were the challenges for you in the workplace?

- What would help you to thrive in the workplace? What would have helped you to thrive?

- What are/were the struggle clashes for you in the workplace? How do you strength nurture in your work?

- What are your safety anchors in the workplace? Are these accommodated? Are these now things that you can feel able to communicate and share?

- If you're considering self-disclosing have you considered the risks involved? Do you feel prepared and supported to self-disclose? Are you clear on what accommodations or adjustments would help you? What do you need to support you in this?

With all the knowledge and understanding that you now have about yourself, you may feel confident in completing the SASA Framework in Chapter 12 and summarizing what it is that you need (accommodations). This tool has assisted many women in enabling and facilitating conversations at work with line managers around accommodations and support needs.

Or it may be that you recognize you need some additional support and guidance. There are a number of organizations, individuals and government support here in the UK such as 'access to work' that may be able to help you, or organizations such as Lexxic and Genius Within, and many individual advocates, coaches and therapists who work from and within the neurodiversity paradigm.

CHAPTER 12

Your Rediscovered Tool Kit

In my rediscovered era

My hope is that this book empowers you on your rediscovered journey, word by word, page by page, chapter by chapter, enabling you to gently explore this brave new world you have been catapulted into. I hope that it is a transformative supporter in the story of rediscovering *you* and a reminder that you are not alone in this journey of coming back to yourself, that you have a guide on this path of late discovery, someone to hold your hand, someone to sit in the dark with you, someone to guide you to the light, and all through a self-affirming, courageous and compassionate lens.

Keep following the light.

Rediscovery is a process, and it's one you have to go 'through' in your own time and in your own way. There are unfortunately no shortcuts or simple ways through. As you find yourself in this new rediscovered world, (which in my mind I imagine an Alaskan beautiful, cold wilderness full of mountains and trees and water and the bluest sky), take the time to gently and curiously explore it. Dip your feet in if you need to until you feel ready, sit with what you are observing, there is no timeline in this new rediscovered world.

Look out for others who are too walking this path into this new world, other wayfinders on their rediscovery journey. These are your people and it makes it a less lonely journey to navigate when you are in the company of others, and community was in my trifecta of tools that very much helped me.

Community is a powerful thing.

Find your community and connect with those who have travelled this road before you. Ask for help when you need it. There are many guides and light givers in this new world who are neuro-inclusive and who will understand and see you and hold space for you as the unravelling unfolds.

I want to leave you with a sense of hope, because hope is the magic anchor we all have access to. Beyond discovery, self-identity and diagnosis, there is a path we all have to walk in this brave new world to finally coming home to yourself.

To rediscovering you.

To finding some peace in your world.

To placing yourself in the centre of your own circle and tuning into your own frequency.

To giving yourself the permission to live and design the life that you have needed all this time.

To being strength focused and struggle aware and supportive.

Look up and around and get self-acquainted with the you of today. Give your present self the attention and compassion you deserve.

Work on finding self-compassion within to honour and respect all the previous versions of you, even the ones you find shameful, painful and deeply horrifying, especially those versions, because they were the ones navigating alone in the dark in your undiscovered world, without self-understanding, access to compassion, or guidance. They deserve a nurturing hug because they are the versions that got the version of you here today as you are reading this.

And on the days when it feels overwhelming, bring yourself back to the here and now, and gently reaffirm to yourself this:

- 'I am coming home to myself.'

- 'I can choose to be kind and accommodating to myself.'

- 'I can be gentle with myself, but also equally the fierce protector and guardian of my frequency, peace and ultimately my health.'

- 'I am giving myself permission to curate the spaces, faces and places that bring me peace, soothe my nervous system and align with my frequency.'

- 'I am worthy and deserving of living my life aligned to my own frequency.'

- 'I am not hard to love.'

- 'It's ok if I find myself sat in the dark depths of this new discovered world, I can extend compassion to myself, I can honour what I'm feeling and why.'

- 'I am enough. I have always been enough.'

Take the time you need.

Pour kindness, love and understanding into yourself and grant yourself the time and the permission to tune into your frequency and savour the stillness that comes from finding your calm on what is an inner self-awakening and self-healing journey.

You are worthy of taking the time you need.

The world will wait for you.

Because whether we take the time or not, the world still keeps on turning around us.

Remind yourself of who you are, where you've been, what you've done, the fear that you've scaled to get here, the courage that has taken, and the light you bring to this rediscovered world.

You found your way here through the dark.

May you find your peace and your people here, and the belonging you need.

Remember that self-permission sits with you. Keep asking yourself what you need and do that thing, however small.

And if asking yourself what you need feels like a hard thing to do, ask yourself what you might need.

What would living my life authentically and aligned to my needs, with the acceptance of who I am and the self-permission to adapt and accommodate my needs look like and change for me?

It's your time to courageously come home to *yourself.*

This is your rediscovered era.

Your rediscovered tool kit

This chapter is your rediscovered tool kit full of four key tried and tested tools that I have developed as part of my own toolkit working with late discovered autistic women that I have referred to throughout the book.

1. The Frequency Circle

2. The SASA Framework

3. The Path of Self-Knowing

4. The Self-Neutrality Concept

1.THE FREQUENCY CIRCLE (THE 12 SS)

This is about putting you at the centre of *your* own circle, tuning into your unique frequency, an alien concept when you've spent your entire life navigating a world that isn't accommodating for the way you experience it. Keeping ourselves safe, ensuring our survival in *that* world has meant employing a safety response that is evolutionary coded into our DNA – the fawning, pleasing, friending in order to keep ourselves safe, or to be seen and not heard. Putting others' needs before our own, hiding our struggles from view, abandoning our own needs, placing us in a constant state of nervous system dysregulation.

If we can trigger a stress response in our bodies, then it makes sense that we can also trigger a relaxation response (our rest and digest state). And when we access and tap into our relaxation response, it's our parasympathetic nervous system that comes into play.

Rather than preparing us for fight or flight, it prepares us for rest. All those physiological symptoms that get ramped up in our stress state get dialled down in our relaxation state – everything from our breathing rate to our blood flow. And it's not just the physiological benefits either – accessing our relaxation response can make us feel better able to cope and it can improve our mood (our prolonged emotional states) and when we are in a better mood, we are much more likely to engage in behaviours that are healthy and self-nurturing, at least in the short term.

We have care labels on clothes and pot plants that tell us what their individual frequency is to thrive and how to care for them, but when it comes to our own understanding, and also being able to articulate that to others in the form of the support and accommodations we need, it's so often lacking. *The Frequency Circle* is your care label for thriving and coming home to yourself. The ultimate barometer test to measure where you are at, how balanced you are within your own frequency circle at any given point in time.

Life is fluid and dynamic and your frequency will need adapting as you navigate through your life to ensure you are at the centre of your own circle, your own world. It's a tool you can use to help navigate your way through burnout and also a tool you can utilize to prevent burnout.

And the power of the frequency circle is that it is person-specific, because we are all unique, and all have differing needs, and it comes with guidance to help you navigate the circle and tune into your own frequency.

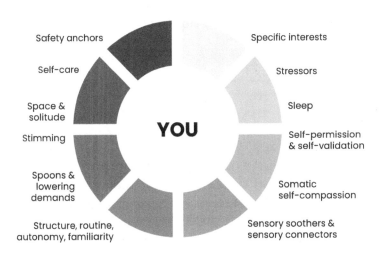

FIGURE 12.1: THE FREQUENCY CIRCLE

Stimming

Stimming is a self-stimulating, repetitive behaviour which serves an important purpose for us when we experience the world in the way that we do. It can help us to self-regulate our emotions, to manage stress and anxiety, to cope with feelings of sensory over or under stimulation, and it can also be something we do that brings us joy or when we are feeling relaxed.

Stims are unique and can be a combination of oral, movement, visual, tactile, auditory based, or they could look like a repetitive activity, or ordering and organizing things.

Up until my late discovery a lot of my stimming was out of sight, hidden from view; nobody would know that I was stimming in their company – even I didn't know that it was stimming. I had no narrative or language to wrap around something that I'd been doing for as long as I could remember, and I discovered many stims that I do that help to regulate and soothe me and tune into my frequency. As part of my developmental history during my autism assessment, I also discovered that my need to order and structure things actually started at a very young age. That fascinated me, how even as a younger version of me I was seeking out ways to soothe my nervous system and interact with the world around me in a way that felt intuitive.

One of those self-soothing stims is to write out the numbers:

- One
- Two
- Six
- Ten

In that order above, written out as words with my finger on my thigh, or sometimes visually in my head with flowing joined up writing. It's something I repeat and repeat and what I discovered when I observed myself was that there was order and flow with these numbers, all having three letters and I find the number three a soothing number, as well as the neat rectangle that is created when the numbers are written out in that order.

I also noticed that whenever I felt anxious I would hold my hands tight in awkward poses and prevent them from moving, or put them out of view in my pockets, especially in certain social situations with people I don't feel safe or comfortable with. So one day I decided to allow myself the freedom to seek out vestibular input in those situations (doing the opposite) and what I discovered was that by allowing myself movement during anxious states, I can find my way back to my frequency.

The flow of movement with a stim toy being twirled around my fingers, some very gentle movement or rocking, or allowing my hands to be animated when I talk brings me home. Needing sensory input is not something to feel ashamed about, it's part of tuning into your needs.

- Do you recognize and understand what your stims are and why they help you?

- What could you learn about your stims if you allowed yourself to observe yourself?

- What would it look and feel like if you gave yourself permission to stim?

Safety anchors

Safety anchors are the things that make *you* feel safe, when your world feels anything but. Tuning into our frequency and feeling regulated means understanding what those safety anchors are. The message we read and hear from people who don't experience the world in the way we do is one of 'self-regulation'. However, co-regulation is an important element of our self-frequency tuning.

That feeling when our storm meets someone's calm and the magic of co-regulation occurs. Fundamentally, co-regulation is about safety and connection, having that person who can provide that consistency and calm when our nervous system has moved into a dysregulated or sympathetic state. We need others to honour our experience.

But we can also become our own safety anchor. When the world feels unsafe, we search for that safety outside of ourselves yet we have an anchor within us that can provide that safety.

- 'I am safe.'

- 'I am my safety anchor.'

- 'Safety resides within me.'

Words that can soothe your nervous system.

Place your hand on your heart and remind yourself that you hold the power.

- Can you identify relationships that provide you with a sense of co-regulation?

- Do you feel safe in your environment (home, work, family, community etc)?

- Who are your safe people and why?

Self-care

'Keeping my body healthy is hard for me. Eating healthy and at appropriate times as well as exercising is a challenge not many who know me see.'

Self-care is about anything and everything we do to take care of ourselves in a way that works for us. It's the relentless endeavours you make, the maintenance measures you take and the safeguarding you put in place to curate a life that feels the way you need it to feel. Even on the hard days. Especially on the hard days. It's the courageous and brave voice that whispers to you to let go of what's not serving you to make way for the new. It's an ongoing process of understanding your needs, giving yourself permission that those needs are valid, deserving and worthy of your energy and your attention, and then taking the action to meet them.

It's asking yourself: 'What do I need today?'

In this moment?

Do that.

Whatever *that* is.

The permission and power sits with you.

- What are the day-to-day things that you do for yourself that help you take care of you?

- What are the things that matter to you?

- What makes self-care difficult?

- What helps you to prioritize self-care?

Structure, routine, autonomy and familiarity

Structure and routines matter and help us tune into our frequency because they minimize our mental load, which is why when we are under stress or in emotional distress you might observe your behaviour becoming even more ordered, routine and repetitive. But that structure and routine needs to be ours, not one that's imposed on us. Autonomy over our day-to-day lives matters, finding a structure that works for us based on where we are at. Structures, order and routines, no matter how small or insignificant they may look from the outside looking in, bring us a sense of predictability to our lives; they help us feel grounded.

- What structures help you?

- What do you struggle with?

- What areas of your life are lacking in the above?

- What are the things/aspects of your life you need to be the same?

- How important is autonomy to you and why?

Somatic self-compassion

'Discovering body/mind centring practices over the past ten years have led me into a deep awareness of my body – its layers of skin, muscle, fascia, bones, organs, nervous system. How these relate to each other and are a one-ness. The signals and sensations which give me a profound awareness of how my body is feeling, balanced or not. So increasingly I connect with the edge of a sensation, can be with it as it settles and does not escalate into overwhelm. This is fundamental to how I currently live my life and continuing autistic revealing.'

Somatic self-compassion is more than just noticing what is happening, it's about being self-attuned, listening in, and working with where you are at. Listening, looking, feeling and connecting to the various parts of your inner body and the signs your body is communicating to you when you are dysregulated and equally when you are tuned into your frequency. Being somatically mindful means asking yourself, 'what am I experiencing right now?' and being somatically compassionate means asking yourself, 'what does my body need right now?'.

The more that we can reconnect with our body, the more compassionate awareness we create which helps us to focus our attention inwards. Create the space and put yourself in the centre of your frequency circle. Dial the noise down and the listening up. That's where self-connection and attunement begin and where somatic self-compassion resides. It's where we dial into our own frequency and where we begin to honour our own needs. Be your own space creator. Commit to wanting to listen somatically.

Your body wants to know that you are the loving, caring guardian and protector committed to helping your body feel safe and there are many ways that you can achieve this through mind work, body work and movement.

- What do you notice?

- How do you connect with yourself somatically?

- How do you signal to your body that you are a safe guardian and protector?

- Where/how do you experience that connection with yourself?

Sleep

When it comes to feeling balanced and in the centre of your own frequency circle then sleep is up there as a top priority and self-compassionate practice. We talked about sleep and our community experiences of sleep back in Chapter 10 so we know how delicate and difficult sleep is for us. Getting a good night's sleep is full of challenges experienced on an individual level. Below are some questions to help you tune into your sleep frequency and to understand your sleep needs more deeply. You are worthy and deserving of nourishing sleep.

- Do you get enough sleep?

- Do you get quality sleep?

- What are your sleep challenges?

- What interferes with your sleep?

- What happens if you don't get enough sleep?

- What helps?

- What's your sleep pattern?

- Do you have a sleep routine?

- What is your natural rhythm? What would it mean to work with that, rather than against it?

- What can you do to aid a more nourishing and compassionate night's sleep?

Specific interests that bring joy (your passions)

'My special interests as a small child were wildly different from other little girls. While others wanted to be a dancer, a nurse or a horse-riding champion, I wanted to be a scuba diver and explorer. I was obsessed with travel, adventure and voyages of discovery. All the books I devoured on these subjects were about men. Sir Ernest Shackleton is one of my heroes and Polar exploration is one of my special interests even today. (I have also discovered stories about pioneering women!)'

We explored passions and the specific interests that bring you joy back in Chapter 5. To further explore how you can tune into your specific interests that bring you joy here are some questions to explore:

- What are your passions and deep interests?

- What brings you joy?

- How can you tune into these more?

- Looking back as a child/young adult what were your passions and deep interests?

- How have they changed over your lifetime?

- What happens when you are unable to access them? Has there been a time in your life when you've not been able to deep dive into your specific interests as much as you need to?

Space and solitude

'Spending too much time together with people, even those whom I love and are extremely important to me is very draining.'

We are space makers and solitude seekers, forever on a quest to find safe places and spaces to retreat to in order to recover from, and take refuge from, the everyday demands in a world that feels too much. The need for deep alone time, recovery and preparation time if we've been around too much sensory input or too many people is where we reset our frequency. From the outside looking in, it might look like an inability to socialize; however, from the inside it's finding our frequency in a world that feels too much.

- What does that look like for you/what do you need?

- How do you carve it out?

- What are the challenges?

- Is your need for space and solitude accommodated?

Stressors (can be sensory, anxiety inducing, demanding, emotional, physical, situational)

There are many neuronormative assumptions you've no doubt heard and have been exposed to that don't take into account the autistic experience, and they sound like this:

- If you expose yourself repeatedly to your stressors, you will eventually 'habituate' to your stressors, and no longer find them distressing.

- You need to 'build resilience' and do more things that you are afraid of.

- You just need to push yourself out of your comfort zone to achieve success.

- You might have grown up being told that you were 'over-reacting' or 'over-responding' to stressors that others didn't find stressful, or punished for your response and were never really 'seen'.

- The more you do them the easier it will be.

- You just need to try harder.

- Nobody else struggles, what's wrong with you?

- I can do this, why can't you?

- Everything is such a big thing for you.

- You are such a drama queen; you always have to make everything about you.

The autistic experience, however, means managing stressors in a different way. Being aware of your stressors means that you are in a better position to manage and minimize their effects, with adaptations that actually support you, rather than placing you in stress response, and with the self-permission to seek out accommodations where you need them. You gain a sense of control over your environment, rather than the environment controlling you.

 ## THE FIVE-STEP SELF-COMPASSIONATE STRESSOR EXERCISE

1. **Identifying** – What are *your* stressors?

2. **Understanding** – Offer yourself some understanding as to why? Why are they stressors for you? Can you RAG them (red, amber, green). What's the struggle underneath the stressor?

3. **Reassuring** – Give yourself some reassurance that your response and your feelings to those stressors are valid and proportionate, rather than dismissing them and your feelings in the process.

4. **Self-knowledge** – Position yourself as the expert on yourself. Ask yourself what do I need? What helps to dial down your stressors? What adaptations do you need? What accommodations would help? Will lowering demands placed on you (from yourself and others) help? Is the juice really worth the squeeze?

5. **Self-permission** – Remind yourself it is ok to have needs. Give yourself the permission to identify what you need. Verbalize what it is that you need. Do that thing that you have identified that you need. Seek out the support or accommodations that you need. Say NO to things.

Sensory soothers, sensory joy givers and sensory connectors

These are all the things that help ground and centre you, that dial up your relaxation (rest and digest) response. All the things that make you feel like you are home. I discovered that there are so many things that help me tune into my frequency and that many are nature-based and elemental. Before my rediscovery, I never really appreciated how much the elements and nature act as both a sensory soother and self-connector.

- Hot baths

- Swimming in (warm) clear blue water

- The sound of water

- An open fire to sit around

- The monochromatic colours in the woods

- Strong sturdy trees to lean on

- Forest bathing

- Blue skies and blue water

- Snow

- Cosy coffee shops

- Flotation tank

- Colourful plant food

- Warm blankets and woolly hats

- Soothing coffee shop jazz

- Vedic meditation

- Kirtan meditation (singing)

- Soundbaths

- Book shops

- Drawing

- Breathwork

- Somatic yoga

- Dressing monochromatic

- Colour (but has to flow and not patterns)

- Scandi design and minimalist interiors

- Deeply connecting with other neurodivergent minds

- What are yours?

- Can you make a list?

- How can you incorporate more of these into your daily life?

- Can you allow yourself to explore more things you've not yet tried?

Spoons and lowering demands

'I recognize how much of the world I do not experience. I could become distraught in allowing this thought to expand and reverberate through my brain. Just now I hold it still within the idea of my window of tolerance. Sparks of where I have been, experiences of the past 15 months – how my window today is more known and conscious and is a very different place to before I was late discovered, and is a very moving place too.

So I hold the thought that I will experience more of the world as my revealing continues. Holding also the deep-felt sense that all that I do now experience is authentic and genuinely me.'

Spoon theory comes from the idea that if you are living with chronic pain, illness, or any condition that causes fatigue then you have less energy on a day-to-day basis to do even the basic everyday tasks. The theory is that you have a certain number of spoons to use in a day, and you need to use them wisely. I discussed how our family uses spoon theory in Chapter 8.

- What are the things that deplete your spoons?

- What are the things that help to replenish them?

- How can you be gentler on yourself?

- What would low demand living look like for you?

Self-permission and self-validation

When we have spent our whole lives asking ourselves *'what's wrong with me?'* and trying harder, our needs repeatedly invalidated and dismissed, it's important to acknowledge the power of self-permission and the compassionate role of self-validation, as you begin to recognize and understand your needs more and more.

The hard bit of this process, however, will be the responses you are so often met with when you start to express those needs. You may have had a lifetime of meeting everyone else's, only to discover yours aren't equally respected.

Part of your rediscovery is making that monumental, self-affirming and courageous shift to 'how does this make me feel?' and 'what do I need?' – listening, and responding and doing in all the ways you need.

Tuning into *your* frequency circle.

2. THE SASA FRAMEWORK

The SASA Framework is a tool I have developed to use in my circle programme and my therapy work. It's a simple, yet effective tool to take all the rediscovered self-knowing you now have and apply it into a framework to help you strength nurture, give your struggles the acceptance they need, to self-advocate and to guide you in asking for what you need.

But don't be fooled by its simplicity.

It takes work to get to a point where you can say 'these are the things I struggle with' and 'these are my strengths; these are the adaptations I am making for myself (the showing up for yourself) and these are the accommodations I need you to support me with.'

And even when we do have that self-knowledge, we hold back on seeking out accommodations or applying the adaptations we need because we don't want to feel like we are a burden or that we've somehow 'failed' because we need support. Often it doesn't feel safe to seek out those accommodations and we can be sensitive to the perceived rejection of our needs – all this on top of the guilt and awkwardness we feel for asking others to help us.

This is a framework that many in our community have used to support self-disclosure at work, particularly when it comes to accommodation requests and to facilitate conversations with loved ones and friends. Understanding both our strengths and struggles, and correlating those to our environment, to people and to how we live our lives, matters in the rediscovered version of you.

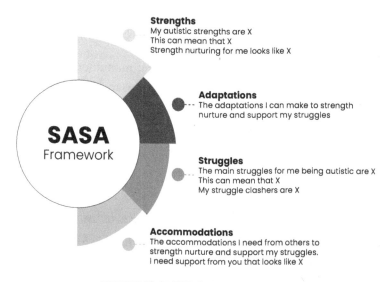

FIGURE 12.2: THE SASA FRAMEWORK

A recent study with autistic people found that those using their strengths often had a better quality of life and wellbeing than those who did not. Strengths-based approaches to autism are increasing in research and clinical practice. Such approaches suggest facilitating autistic people to increase the use of their strengths leads to positive outcomes (e.g. improved wellbeing). However, autistic people report less knowledge and use of their strengths compared to neurotypicals (Taylor *et al.*, 2023).

3. THE PATH OF SELF-KNOWING (MELTDOWNS/SHUTDOWNS/OVERSPILLS)

A 'path of self-knowing' exercise to guide you in forensically examining and understanding your meltdown and shutdown experiences.

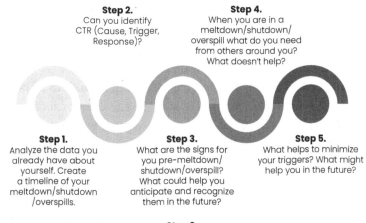

Step 2.
Can you identify CTR (Cause, Trigger, Response)?

Step 4.
When you are in a meltdown/shutdown/overspill what do you need from others around you? What doesn't help?

Step 1.
Analyze the data you already have about yourself. Create a timeline of your meltdown/shutdown /overspills.

Step 3.
What are the signs for you pre-meltdown/shutdown/overspill? What could help you anticipate and recognize them in the future?

Step 5.
What helps to minimize your triggers? What might help you in the future?

Step 6.
What helps post-meltdown/shutdown/overspill? What do you need? What can you learn from them to better understand your needs?

FIGURE 12.3: THE PATH OF SELF-KNOWING

4. THE SELF-NEUTRALITY CONCEPT

We are surrounded with messages of 'Love yourself more'.

Indeed, in this book you've heard me say: 'Show yourself compassion' and 'Be more accepting of yourself and more compassionately aware.'

But when we struggle with low self-worth, we can feel like we are always on the periphery of self-love, kindness, acceptance and compassion, and what happens is that self-criticism, negative self-talk, self-invalidation and self-dismissal become our default norm.

Somewhere in the middle lies the concept of self-neutrality.

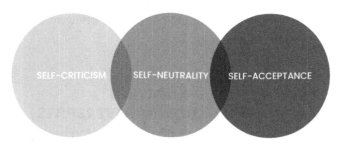

FIGURE 12.4: THE SELF-NEUTRALITY CONCEPT

It's the middle ground – neither completely positively self-affirming, but not destructively negative either. It's a starting point if you are struggling with that shift towards more positive and nurturing self-talk and ultimately the self-practice of compassion.

It might look like, as a first step, allowing yourself to be more observant of yourself in times of struggle and emotional distress, and taking a more neutral or centred position towards yourself, a step away from the gravitational pull that is apathy, and a step closer towards the light that is eventual compassion.

When your inner narrative feels stuck in that place where you believe that you are not deserving of love, compassion and acceptance, start by finding some middle ground, rather than the default position of self-criticism you automatically go to.

It might sound like:

- 'I am a human being, and all human beings deserve to be loved and to feel a sense of belonging.'

- 'I am working on finding acceptance of myself.'

- 'We are all a work in progress.'

- 'I am in the process of rediscovering myself.'

Self-neutrality is a middle ground that with practice, can lead you to a more gradual shift in the right direction on your journey towards more self-compassion.

Conclusion

The end of this book marks a new beginning in the story of you. Because when we have lived a lifetime of being *undiscovered* our nervous systems have, up until now, already been through so much. The closing of this book marks the beginning of your rediscovered era, the next chapter in your story which is about finding your frequency, and tuning into that, putting your whole self fully in the centre of your circle for what might be the first time.

Soothing and nurturing yourself with deep loving breaths, self-permission and the compassionate and courageous practices that you can hopefully now see fill you with a sense of calm and peace.

We are all a work in progress, and we are constantly evolving and learning, nothing stands still or stays the same and that is true about what standing in the centre of your circle looks like. It's a daily practice from here on in of being compassionate and courageous, standing proud in the centre of your circle, and being the fierce guardian and protector of your energy, your peace and your world.

You are worthy and deserving of that stillness and peace that comes from being in the middle of your own frequency circle.

Even on the days when it feels hard, and when your default slips back into the 'no needs' version of you, and you momentarily step outside of your frequency circle and into other people's circles, because that's where it feels safest for you in that moment – ultimately because that is how you've survived in a world that isn't built for the way you experience it.

Hold that compassionate self-awareness you are worthy of, without the self-judgement. Acknowledge and recognize why you are outside of your own circle, and what you need to help you get back home to your own.

This book is called a *compassionate and courageous guide* because I see the depth of courage it takes to go on this journey of rediscovery, the othering and the detachment it creates (from your sense of self and how others see and experience you) as you shift yourself from one world into another. I see the compassion you have to extend to yourself in the process.

And the really helpful thing about compassion is that it allows us to extend kindness and understanding towards ourselves even in times of struggle without being self-critical. It allows us to mindfully connect the dots without being judgemental, and it enables a sense of self-connectedness reminding us that we are only human in those moments and on those days when things feel too hard. There is no space for toxic positivity or self-invalidation.

It allows you to be you.

And in the midst of struggle, and all the future mountains you will climb in this new rediscovered world, look for the light. Embody its power and strength. Honouring your struggle *and* embodying the light can co-exist too.

You're not alone in this.

You belong here.

Put your hand on your heart and feel the energy of that sense of belonging through these pages and words.

Be proud of the rediscovered version of you.

Be proud of all the versions of you.

I want to leave you with the knowledge that your rediscovery is a profound milestone in the story of you, because you have not only opened the door to a brave new world, you've also birthed a new version of you and I know that your self-understanding and self-knowing is only going to grow and expand from here.

With love and compassion,

Catherine Asta x

References

Chapter 1

Lavender, J. (2021). *Why Meditate? Because It Works*. London: Hodder & Stoughton.

The London Meditation Centre. (2024). What is Vedic Meditation? www.londonmeditationcentre.com

Sequeria, S. & Ahmed, M. (2012, June). Meditation as a potential therapy for autism: A review. *PubMed*. 10.1155/2012/835847

Chapter 2

Alyward, B.S., Gal-Szabo, D.E. & Taraman, S. (2021, September). Racial, Ethnic, and Sociodemographic Disparities in Diagnosis of Children with Autism Spectrum Disorder. *PubMed Central*. 10.1097/DBP.0000000000000996

Bouzy, J., Brunelle, J., Cohen, D. & Condat, A. (2023, May). Transidentities and autism spectrum disorder: A systematic review. *Elsevier*. https://doi.org/10.1016/j.psychres.2023.115176

Cazalis, F. (2022, April). Evidence that nine autistic women out of ten have been victims of sexual violence. *PubMed*. http://dx.doi.org/10.3389/fnbeh.2022.852203

Davies, J., Cooper, K., Killick, E., Sam, E., Healy, M., Thompson, G. & Kane, L. (2024, February). Autistic identity: A systematic review of quantitative research. *PubMed*. Retrieved May 23, 2024, from https://pubmed.ncbi.nlm.nih.gov/38334318

Diemer, M.C. & Regester, A. (2022, July). Autism presentation in female and Black populations: Examining the roles of identity, theory, and systemic inequalities. *Research Gate*. 10.1177/13623613221113501

D'Mello, A.M., Frosch, I.R., Li, C.E., Cardinaux, A.L. & Gabrielli, J.D. (2022, August). Exclusion of females in autism research: Empirical evidence for a 'leaky' recruitment-to-research pipeline. *Wiley*. doi.org/10.1002/aur.2795

Estrin, G., Milner, V., Spain, D., Happé, F. & Colvert, E. (2020, October). Barriers to autism spectrum disorder diagnosis for young women and girls: A systematic review. *PubMed*. Retrieved May 23, 2024, from https://pubmed. ncbi.nlm.nih.gov/34868805.

Happé, F., Rumball, F. & Grey, N. (2020, December). Experience of trauma and PTSD symptoms in autistic adults: Risk of PTSD development following DSM-5 and non-DSM-5 traumatic life events. *PubMed*. 10.1002/aur.2306

Kallitsounaki, A., Williams, D.M. & Lind, S.E. (2021). Links between autistic traits, feelings of gender dysphoria, and mentalising ability: Replication and extension of previous findings from the general population. *Springer*. 10.1007/s10803-020-04626-w

Loomes, R., Hull, L., Polmear, W. & Locke, M. (2017, June). What is the male-to-female ratio in autism spectrum Disorder? A systematic review and meta-analysis. *PubMed*. 10.1016/j.jaac.2017.03.013

Moseley, R.L., Druce, T. & Turner-Cobb, J.M. (2020, January 31). 'When my autism broke': A qualitative study spotlighting autistic voices on menopause. *NCBI*. Retrieved May 23, 2024, from https://www.ncbi.nlm.nih.gov/pmc/articles/PMC7376624/

NHS England. (2023, December 12). *Meeting the needs of autistic adults in mental health services*. NHS England. Retrieved May 23, 2024, from www.england.nhs.uk/publication/meeting-the-needs-of-autistic-adults-in-mental-health-services

ONS. (2021, February 19). *New shocking data highlights the autism employment gap*. National Autistic Society. Retrieved May 23, 2024, from www.autism.org.uk/what-we-do/news/new-data-on-the-autism-employment-gap

Pavlopoulou, G. & Dimitriou, D. (2018, August 7). *Autistic adults and sleep problems*. National Autistic Society. Retrieved May 23, 2024, from https://www.autism.org.uk/advice-and-guidance/professional-practice/sleep-adults

Pearson, A., Rees, J. & Forster, S. (2022, June). 'This was just how this friendship worked': Experiences of interpersonal victimization among autistic adults. *PubMed*. 10.1089/aut.2021.0035

Ward, J.H., Weir, E., Allison, C. & Baron-Cohen, S. (2023, September). Increased rates of chronic physical health conditions across all organ systems in autistic adolescents and adults. *Molecular Autism*. https://doi.org/10.1186/s13229-023-00565-2

Chapter 3

Harris, A., Katzman, D., Norris, M. & Zucker, N. (2019, October). Avoidant Restrictive Food Intake and ASD. *Journal of the American Academy of Child & Adolescent Psychiatry*. https://doi.org/10.1016/j.jaac.2019.08.072

Inouye, T., Otani, R., Igutchi, T. & Ishii, R. (2021, May). Prevalence of autism spectrum disorder and autistic traits in children with anorexia nervosa and avoidant/restrictive food intake disorder. *BioPsychoSocial Medicine*. https://doi.org/10.1186/s13030-021-00212-3

Trevisan, D., Parker, T. & McPartland, J. (2021, October). First-hand accounts of interoceptive difficulties in autistic adults. *National Library of Medicine*. 10.1007/s10803-020-04811-x

Chapter 4

Kinnaird, E., Stewart, C. & Tchanturia, K. (2020, January). Investigating alexithymia in autism: A systematic review and meta-analysis. *Cambridge Core.*

Chapter 5

Adkin, T. & Gray, D. (2022, July 14). *Guest Post: What is monotropic split?* Emergent Divergence. Retrieved May 24, 2024, from https://emergentdivergence.com/2022/07/14/guest-post-what-is-monotropic-split

American Psychiatric Association. DSM-5 Task Force. (2017). *Diagnostic and Statistical Manual of Mental Disorders: DSM-5.* CBS Publishers & Distributors, Pvt. Limited.

Murray, D., Lawson, W. & Lesser, M. (2005, May). Attention, monotropism and the diagnostic criteria for autism. *Sage.* doi.org/10.1177/1362361305051398

Chapter 6

ARI. (2024). Autism Research Institute. Retrieved May 30, 2024, from https://autism.org/meltdowns-calming-techniques-in-autism

NHS England. (2023) Meeting the needs of autistic adults in mental health services - guidance for integrated care boards, health organisations and w. (2023). NHS England. Retrieved May 30, 2024, from www.england.nhs.uk/wp-content/uploads/2023/12/B1800-meeting-the-needs-of-autistic-adults-in-mental-health-services.pdf

NAS. (2024). www.autism.org.uk

O'Connor, R. (2021). *When It Is Darkest: Why People Die by Suicide and What We Can Do to Prevent It.* London: Random House UK.

Supekar, K., Uddin, L., Khousam, A., Phillips, J., Gaillard, W., Kenworthy, L., Yerys, B. & Menon, V. (2013). Brain hyper-connectivity in children with autism and its links to social deficits. *National Library of Medicine.* 10.1016/j.celrep.2013.10.001

Chapter 7

Arnold, S., Higgins, J., Weise, J., Desai, A., Pellicano, E. & Trollor, J. (2023, October). Confirming the nature of autistic burnout. *National Library of Medicine.* 10.1177/13623613221147410

Kim, J. & Kim, E. (2023, February). Neurocognitive effects of stress: a metaparadigm perspective. *National Library of Medicine.* 10.1038/s41380-023-01986-4

Klopack, E., Crimmins, E., Cole, S. & Carroll, J. (2022, April). Social stressors associated with age-related T lymphocyte percentages in older US adults: Evidence from the US Health and Retirement Study. *PNAS.* https://doi.org/10.1073/pnas.2202780119

Chapter 8

Pearson, A. & Rose, K. (2023). *Autistic Masking: Understanding Identity Management and the Role of Stigma*. Shoreham-by-Sea: Pavilion Publishing & Media Limited.

Chapter 9

Cazalis, F., Reyes, E., Leduc, S. & Gourion, D. (2022, April). Evidence that nine autistic women out of ten have been victims of sexual violence. *National Library of Medicine*. https://pubmed.ncbi.nlm.nih.gov/35558435/

Milton, D. (2012, June). On the ontological status of autism: The 'double empathy problem'. *Taylor & Francis*. https://doi.org/10.1080/09687599.2012.710008

Pearson, A., Rees, J. & Forster, S. (2022, June). 'This was just how this friendship worked': Experiences of interpersonal victimization among autistic adults. *National Library of Medicine*. https://pubmed.ncbi.nlm.nih.gov/36605970/

Tripp, J.C. & McDevitt-Murphy, M.E. (2017). Trauma related guilt mediates the relationship between posttraumatic stress disorder and suicidal ideation. *Suicide and Life Threatening Behaviour, 4791*, 78–85. https://doi.org/10.1111/sltb.12266

Chapter 10

Baeza-Velasco, C., Cohen, C., Hamonet, D., Vlamynck, C. *et al.* (2018, December). Autism, joint hypermobility-related disorders and pain. *National Library of Medicine*. 10.3389/fpsyt.2018.00656

Besag, F. (2018, December). Epilepsy in patients with autism: links, risks and treatment challenges. *National Library of Medicine*. 10.2147/NDT.S120509

Cassidy, S., Au-Yeung, S. & Robertson, A. (2022, February). Autism and autistic traits in those who died by suicide in England. *Cambridge University Press*. doi:10.1192/bjp.2022.21

Clapp, I., Paul, K., Beck, E. & Nho, S. (2021, March). Hypermobile disorders and their effects on the hip joint. *National Library Of Medicine*. 10.3389/fsurg.2021.596971

Hall, A., Maw, R., Illes-Caven, Y., Gregory, S., Rai, D. & Golding, J. (2023, February). Associations between autistic traits and early ear and upper respiratory signs: a prospective observational study of the Avon Longitudinal Study of Parents and Children (ALSPAC) geographically defined childhood population. *BMJ Open*. 10.1136/bmjopen-2022-067682

Happé, F., Rumball, F. & Grey, N. (2020, April). Experience of trauma and PTSD Symptoms in autistic adults: Risk of PTSD development following DSM-5 and non-DSM-5 traumatic life events. *National Library of Medicine*. 10.1002/aur.2306

Haruvi-Lamdan, N., Horesh, S.Z., Kraus, M. & Golan, O. (2020). Autism spectrum disorder and post-traumatic stress disorder: An unexplored co-occurence of conditions. *Autism* 24(4), 884–898.

Kirby, A., Connor, C. & Mazefsky, C. (2024, February). Are autistic females at greater risk of suicide? A call for clarity to advance suicide prevention for the whole community. *Wiley Online Library*. https://doi.org/10.1002/aur.3120

Moseley, R., Druce, T. & Turner-Cobb, J. (2020, August). 'When my autism broke': A qualitative study spotlighting autistic voices on menopause. *National Library of Medicine*. 10.1177/1362361319901184

NHS England. (2023). *Meeting the needs of autistic adults in mental health services – guidance for integrated care boards, health organisations and wider system partners*. (2023). NHS England. Retrieved May 30, 2024, from www.england.nhs.uk/wp-content/uploads/2023/12/B1800-meeting-the-needs-of-autistic-adults-in-mental-health-services.pdf

Steenfeldt-Kristensen, C., Jones, C.A. & Richards, C. (2020) The prevalence of self-injurious behaviour in autism: A meta-analytic study. *Journal of Autism & Developmental Disorders, 50*, 3857–3873. https://doi.org/10.1007/s10803-020-04443-1

Chapter 12

Taylor, E., Livingston, L. & Shah, P. (2023, January). Psychological strengths and well-being: Strengths use predicts quality of life, well-being and mental health in autism. *Sage*.